Cancer Treatment and Research

Volume 181

Series Editor

Steven T. Rosen, Duarte, CA, USA

This book series provides detailed updates on the state of the art in the treatment of different forms of cancer and also covers a wide spectrum of topics of current research interest. Clinicians will benefit from expert analysis of both standard treatment options and the latest therapeutic innovations and from provision of clear guidance on the management of clinical challenges in daily practice. The research-oriented volumes focus on aspects ranging from advances in basic science through to new treatment tools and evaluation of treatment safety and efficacy. Each volume is edited and authored by leading authorities in the topic under consideration. In providing cutting-edge information on cancer treatment and research, the series will appeal to a wide and interdisciplinary readership. The series is listed in PubMed/Index Medicus.

More information about this series at http://www.springer.com/series/5808

Vinod Pullarkat • Guido Marcucci
Editors

Biology and Treatment of Leukemia and Bone Marrow Neoplasms

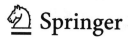 Springer

Editors
Vinod Pullarkat
Department of Hematology and
Hematopoietic Cell Transplantation
Gehr Family Center for Leukemia Research
Duarte, CA, USA

Guido Marcucci
Department of Hematology and
Hematopoietic Cell Transplantation
Gehr Family Center for Leukemia Research
Duarte, CA, USA

ISSN 0927-3042   ISSN 2509-8497   (electronic)
Cancer Treatment and Research
ISBN 978-3-030-78313-6   ISBN 978-3-030-78311-2   (eBook)
https://doi.org/10.1007/978-3-030-78311-2

This Springer imprint is published by the registered company Springer Nature Switzerland AG
The registered company address is: Gewerbestrasse 11, 6330 Cham, Switzerland

Introduction

Our understanding of the biology and treatment of acute leukemias and other bone marrow neoplasms is evolving rapidly. Advances in genomics and sequencing technology over the last decade have made genetic analysis of these disorders accessible to practicing clinicians, thereby aiding in more accurate diagnosis as well as risk stratification of these disorders. The development of novel therapies for bone marrow neoplasms is also advancing at a rapid pace with many novel highly active agents approved recently. Given these advances, it is all the more important that comprehensive diagnostic work up is performed up front so that the most appropriate therapy can be chosen. In this volume, using real-life case scenarios, the authors, each of whom is an expert in their field, describe how modern diagnostic testing and work up translates into accurate prognostication and aids in the choice of therapy for bone marrow neoplasms.

Use of next generation sequencing to evaluate blood cytopenias has led to increasing detection of clonal hematopoiesis particularly in older individuals. This finding has various implications for patients including evolution to myeloid malignancies like myelodysplastic syndrome (MDS) and acute myeloid leukemia (AML). In Chap. 1, the authors describe the evaluation and classification of clonal cytopenias, MDS and AML and discuss prognostic implication of genetic findings. Therapy of MDS including novel agents in development is discussed in Chap. 7.

Although acute lymphoblastic leukemia (ALL) is eminently curable in over 90% of children, adults will this disease do not have the same favorable outcome, largely in part due to adverse genetic features of their leukemia. This is particularly true for Philadelphia-like ALL, a poor prognostic entity that is fairly common among adults, but difficult to diagnose. Chapter 2 discusses in detail how advances in genomic sequencing and diagnostic technology apply to accurate prognostication of ALL and can aid in judicious application of potentially curative therapies like allogeneic hematopoietic cell transplantation (alloHCT). Treatment of ALL has been transformed by development of immunotherapies that are highly active in this disease. These include bispecific antibodies, immunoconjugates as well as chimeric antigen receptor modified T (CAR-T) cells. These therapies allow relapsed refractory patients a high chance of achieving a deep remission enabling them to undergo potentially curative alloHCT. Therapy of ALL is discussed in Chap. 5 and CAR-T cell therapy is covered in Chap. 11.

The treatment of acute promyelocytic leukemia (APL) is a triumph of modern oncology and has transformed a uniformly fatal disease to one that is almost always curable nowadays if accurate diagnosis is made early. More importantly, most patients at the present time can be cured with a regimen that avoids conventional chemotherapy. Advances in the treatment of APL are discussed in Chap. 3. The treatment of AML has seen dramatic change over the last 5 years or so after decades of minimal progress. Multiple highly active novel agents like the Bcl-2 inhibitor venetoclax have been approved in recent years thereby expanding the options available for patients, particularly older adults who still have a poor long-term outcome with current therapies due to comorbidities and adverse genetics. Treatment of AML including data on novel therapies is covered in Chap. 4.

The development of the tyrosine kinase inhibitor imatinib for therapy of chronic myeloid leukemia (CML) ushered a revolution in targeted therapy for hematologic neoplasms. Since then multiple new TKIs have been developed for CML and have resulted in excellent quality of life and normal life expectancy for most patients affected by this leukemia. CML therapy is the subject of Chap. 6. Chronic lymphocytic leukemia (CLL) is the commonest leukemia in the western world and affects older adults. Until recently treatments for CLL were chemotherapy based and were poorly tolerated by older patients. However recent years have witnessed a dramatic transformation in treatment of CLL with development of BTK inhibitors, Bcl-2 inhibitors as well as anti CD20 antibodies. Most patients currently can be spared chemotherapy and enjoy durable long-term remissions Therapy of CLL is discussed in Chap. 8.

Our understanding of the biology myeloproliferative neoplasms MPN) has seen major advances with identification of mutations that lead to MPN. However, the novel therapies do not alter disease course or progression to bone marrow fibrosis and alloHCT remains the only curative option for suitable patients. Therefore, prognostication of the disorders is critical for preventing transformation to AML and permits optimal timing of potentially toxic therapies like alloHCT. These issues are discussed in Chap. 9. Systemic mastocytosis (SM) is a rare entity that can be indolent or aggressive, the latter carrying a poor prognosis. Treatment for SM has been unsatisfactory, particularly for cases associated with another hematologic neoplasm. However, novel therapies for SM are being developed and offer promise for this difficult to treat disorder. Biology and treatment of SM is discussed in Chap. 10.

In summary, therapy of leukemias and other bone marrow neoplasms has witnessed a dramatic transformation in the last decade and hopefully such rapid progress will continue, thereby improving the survival and quality of life of patients. We have attempted to summarize a large volume of recent data into a concise volume that will be a useful guide for day-to-day patient management. We hope this volume will be a valuable resource to students of hematologic malignancies as well as practicing physicians alike.

Vinod Pullarkat, MD, MRCP
Guido Marcucci, MD

Contents

Advances in Diagnosis and Risk Stratification of Acute Myeloid Leukemia and Myelodysplastic Syndromes

1

Raju K. Pillai and Michelle Afkhami

Contents

1.1 Next Generation Sequencing (NGS)- Based Testing in Hematologic Malignancies

Advances in NGS triggered by the human genome project have enabled genomic profiling of hematopoietic malignancies in routine clinical practice. In comparison to traditional methods like Sanger sequencing, NGS technology enables sequencing

R. K. Pillai (✉) · M. Afkhami
City of Hope Medical Center, 1500 E Duarte Rd, Duarte, CA 91010, USA
e-mail: rpillai@coh.org

© Springer Nature Switzerland AG 2021
V. Pullarkat and G. Marcucci (eds.), *Biology and Treatment of Leukemia and Bone Marrow Neoplasms*, Cancer Treatment and Research 181,
https://doi.org/10.1007/978-3-030-78311-2_1

Fig. 1.1 Sequential steps for analysis of a peripheral blood or bone marrow sample for detection of clinically significant genomic alterations

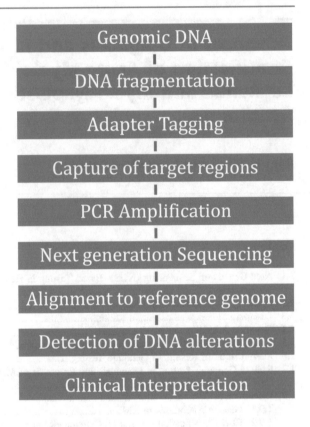

Genomic DNA

DNA fragmentation

Adapter Tagging

Capture of target regions

PCR Amplification

Next generation Sequencing

Alignment to reference genome

Detection of DNA alterations

Clinical Interpretation

billions of DNA molecules in a massively parallel fashion which significantly reduces cost. The cost of sequencing the whole genome is now approaching $1000 and is expected to decline further. Most laboratories sequence targeted genes (gene panels) for clinical practice, but exome sequencing is becoming widely available. All these assays can be performed from bone marrow aspirates or peripheral blood samples collected in EDTA.

Sample preparation begins with DNA fragmentation using physical shearing or enzymatic digestion to yield fragments of desired length (Fig. 1.1). Fragments from regions of interest are enriched by hybridization using target baits or by using PCR-based methods. Adapters are now added to the enriched fragments to create a library for sequencing. Sequencing data comprising the sequence of the DNA fragments with quality information (FASTQ files) are now aligned to the human genome using bioinformatics software to detect DNA alterations including single nucleotide variants (SNV) and insertions/deletions (indels) which are typically stored in a variant call format file (VCF file). Copy number variations (CNV) can also be identified from the sequencing data using specialized software.

Variants detected are matched against databases of normal variants in the population (eg. ExAC, gnomAD) as well as databases of tumor-associated variants (eg. COSMIC). Variants are classified as pathogenic, likely pathogenic, variant of unknown significance, likely benign or benign based on allele frequency in the normal population, effect on protein structure and function, in silico prediction algorithms, and other evidence available in the literature.

RNA sequencing can be accomplished using a similar process that includes initial conversion of mRNA to cDNA. RNA sequencing is more sensitive for detection of structural variants such as gene fusions. RNA sequencing also enables gene expression profiling and assessment of pathway activation. Epigenetic alterations play an important role in the pathogenesis of myelodysplastic syndrome (MDS) and acute myeloid leukemia (AML). The primary epigenetic alterations include methylation of the cytosine nucleotide as well as modifications of histone proteins. DNA methylation can be assessed by NGS, but these methods are not routinely available in the clinical laboratory. The following sections will describe the application of DNA sequencing using a targeted panel for patient management.

1.2 CASE 1: 69 Year Old with Pancytopenia

An asymptomatic 69-year-old male had pancytopenia detected on a routine complete blood count. A subsequent bone marrow examination showed a mildly hypercellular marrow for age (50%) with multilineage dyspoietic changes without increase in blasts. Conventional cytogenetic studies revealed a normal male karyotype. Per WHO 2016 criteria, a diagnosis of myelodysplastic syndrome requires sustained cytopenia and at least one of the 3 following criteria—morphologic dysplasia in > 10% of one or more hematopoietic lineages, clonal cytogenetic abnormality excluding those that are AML defining or increased blasts (>5%). The patient was diagnosed with myelodysplastic syndrome (MDS) with multilineage dysplasia. Targeted sequencing studies were performed using a NGS- based panel. The results are shown in Table 1.1. Bone marrow evaluation after 12 months of 5-azacytidine therapy showed progression of disease with increase in blasts to 15%. He was started on combination therapy with 5-azacytidine and venetoclax and underwent a matched unrelated donor hematopoietic stem cell transplantation.

Table 1.1 Results of NGS-based mutation testing from bone marrow aspirate

Gene	Alteration	Allele Frequency (%)
ASXL1	c.1934dup; p.G646Wfs*12	43
NRAS	c.38G > T; p.G13V	14
RUNX1	c.602G > A; p.R201Q	32
STAG2	c.328C > T; p.R110*	33
TET2	c.3409 + 2_3409 + 3insT	30
TET2	c.3661 T > C; p.C1221R	33

1.3 Discussion

This case highlights several important questions about the role of genetic profiling in the pathogenesis, risk stratification, and management of MDS. Myelodysplastic syndromes include a heterogeneous group of clonal disorders characterized by dyspoietic cytomorphology, ineffective hematopoiesis, and cytopenias with eventual transformation into acute myeloid leukemia (AML) in the majority of patients. With the advent of cost-effective NGS technologies, the genomic alterations in MDS have now been extensively characterized. However, these are not yet used for prognostication in the International prognostic scoring system (IPSS).

Table 1.2 Recurrent cytogenetic abnormalities detected in myelodysplastic syndrome

CNV (Losses)	CNV (Gains)	Translocations
− 7 or del(7q)	+ 6	t(3;3)(q21;q26)
− 5 or del(5q)	+ 8*	inv3(q21q26)
del(9q)	+ 21	t(3;21)(q26;q22)
del(11q)		t(1;7)(p11;p11)
del(12p)		t(2;11)(p21;q23)
− 13 or del(13q)		t(11;16)(q23;p13)
− 17, i(17q)		t(6;9)(p23;q34)
− 20 or del(20q)*		t(2;11)(p21;q23)
- 21		unbalanced translocations at 17p
-Y*		unbalanced translocations at 12p

* Not used for diagnosis since these abnormalities can be seen in older age group and non-MDS entities

Table 1.3 Major pathways and driver genes in MDS

Pathway/functions	Driver genes
DNA methylation	*DNMT3A, TET2, IDH1, IDH2, WT1*
Chromatin modification	*EZH2, SUZ12, ASXL1, KMT2, KDM6A, ARID2, PHF6, ATRX*
RNA splicing	*SF3B1, SRSF2, U2AF1, ZRSR2, PRPF8*
Cohesin complex	*STAG1, STAG2, RAD21, SMC3, SMC1A*
Transcription	*RUNX1, ETV6, GATA2, CEBPA, BCOR, BCORL1, SETBP1, MECOM*
Cytokine receptor/tyrosine kinase	*FLT3, KIT, JAK2, MPL, CALR, CSF3R, NRAS, KRAS, CBL, PTPN11, GNAS*
Checkpoint/cell cycle	*TP53, CDKN2A*
DNA repair	*ATM, BRCC3, FANCL*
Others	*NPM1, DDX41*

1.4   Genomic Alterations in MDS

Cytogenetic abnormalities are seen in about 50–60% of MDS diagnostic specimens. The major recurrent abnormalities are summarized in Table 1.2. Gain or loss of chromosomal segments are the most common abnormalities seen [1]. Recurrent translocations are less common and include unbalanced translocations, which may lead to loss of gain of genetic material.

Genomic profiling has shown that the pathogenesis of MDS is related to sequential acquisition of mutations in a group of genes involved in hematopoiesis. Most MDS samples display about 9 somatic mutations within the coding sequence including both driver and nondriver mutations [2]. The major pathways and genes that are involved in the pathogenesis of MDS are shown in Table 1.3 [2, 3]. The major functional pathways include RNA splicing, DNA methylation, transcription, chromatin modification, signal transduction, DNA repair, and other pathways (Table 1.3). The most common mutated genes in MDS include those involved in DNA methylation (*TET2, DNMT3A, and IDH1/2*), chromatin modification (*ASXL1, EZH2, MLL2*), transcriptional regulation (*RUNX1, TP53*), signal transduction (*NRAS, KRAS*), and RNA splicing (*SF3B1, SRSF2, U2AF1, U2AF2*) [4–8] (Fig. 1.1).

1.5   Clonal Hematopoiesis of Indeterminate Potential and Pathogenesis of MDS

Many of the MDS associated mutations described above have been detected in apparently healthy individuals and are therefore not diagnostic of MDS in isolation. Hematopoietic stem cells (HSC) replace an estimated 10^{10}–10^{12} cells daily [9]. Since HSC are reported to acquire one coding mutation for a decade of life, the HSC population in older adults are essentially somatic genetic mosaics [10]. Mutations that confer a proliferative advantage leads to generation of a clonal population of cells. Clonal Hematopoiesis (CH) has been defined as the expansion of one lineage of cells at a rate disproportionate to other clones [3]. CH is common in elderly population and is estimated to be detectable in up to 30% of subjects over 60 years [3, 11]. The most frequently mutated genes are DNMT3A, TET2, and ASXL1.

Table 1.4 Relationship between CH, CHIP, CCUS, and MDS

Feature	CH	CHIP	CCUS	MDS
Clonal population	+	+	+	+
Dyspoiesis	±	-	-	±
Cytopenia	±	-	+	+
Recurrent genetic abnormalities	±	-	-	±

Clonal hematopoiesis of indeterminate potential (CHIP) refers to the presence of a clonal population with somatic mutations with at least a 2% variant allele frequency involving a known driver of hematopoietic neoplasms [12]. In contrast, clonal cytopenia of undetermined significance (CCUS) are associated with CH and cytopenias [12, 13] but no morphologic dysplasia (Table 1.4).

Both CHIP and MDS have a strong association with increasing age and have overlapping genes that are mutated and are likely to share similar pathogenetic mechanisms. MDS is more advanced with significantly different clinical implications. In contrast, patients diagnosed with MDS will have dyspoiesis greater than 10% of cells in at least one of the 3 lineages in the bone marrow or will have a clonal population with an MDS defining karyotype. The yearly rate of progression from CHIP to leukemia is approximately 1% whereas the risk is much higher in MDS. The vast majority of CHIP cases have a single mutation whereas MDS typically has several [12]. CHIP is associated with much longer survival and medical intervention is not recommended. CHIP however is associated with increased risk of cardiovascular disease [11].

1.6   Interpretation of Results of Genomic Testing

The implications of the genomic alterations seen in this patient are discussed below in the context of gene function and the effects on protein structure and function. Variants are classified as pathogenic, likely pathogenic, variant of unknown significance, likely benign or benign based on allele frequency in the normal population, effect on protein structure and function, in silico prediction algorithms, and other evidence available in the literature.

A frameshift alteration at codon 646 of the *ASXL1* gene was detected. The p. G646Wfs*12 frameshift mutation detected in this patient is the most commonly recurrent alteration of *ASXL1*, and frameshift alterations are expected to cause premature termination and likely loss of function of the gene. Mutations in ASXL1 are associated with an adverse prognosis [14].

A missense alteration at codon 13 of the *NRAS* gene was detected. The RAS proteins regulate signal transduction upon binding of ligand to a variety of membrane receptors. *RAS* gene mutations at codons 12, 13, and 61 confer constitutive activation of the RAS protein. The activating mutations in the *NRAS* gene have been implicated in the differentiation of progenitor cells into leukemic cells [15].

A missense alteration at codon 201 of the RUNX1 gene was detected. The RUNX1 gene encodes the DNA binding unit of the heterodimeric CBF that is a critical regulator of definitive hematopoiesis. The RUNX1 mutations are commonly detected in MDS and acute myeloid leukemia (AML) and associated with poor prognosis [16]. The p.R201Q mutation detected in this specimen has been previously reported in patients with AML.

A nonsense alteration at codon 110 of the STAG2 gene was detected. The STAG2 gene encodes a component of the cohesin complex that participates in the regulation of sister chromatid separation during mitosis. Mutations of the STAG2 gene have been found in approximately 6% of MDS and 1–2% of AML. The p. R110* frameshift mutation detected in this patient has been reported in patients with AML, and frameshift alterations are expected to cause premature termination and likely loss of function of the gene.

An insertion of T between nucleotides c.3409 + 2 and 3409 + 3 and a missense alteration at codon 1221 of the TET2 gene were detected. TET2 mutations are frequently found in myeloid cancers and generally result in loss of function. The c.3409 + 2_3409 + 3insT alteration is close to the donor splice site of exon 3, and analysis of this alteration using multiple in silico tools predicts that the splice site at this position would be obliterated, which is likely to result in loss of function. The p. C1221R alteration detected in this patient has been previously reported in patients with myeloid neoplasms.

1.7 Role of Genomic Testing in Diagnosis and Prognosis of MDS

Although detection of genetic abnormalities in MDS is useful for establishing a clonal process, identification of MDS type mutations, even in the presence of cytopenias, should not be used per WHO 2016 criteria, to establish a diagnosis of MDS if there is no morphologic dysplasia. The role of these mutations in determining prognosis, either alone or in combination, is currently under intense investigation. However, molecular alterations are not used in current prognostic scoring systems such as the International Prognostic Scoring System (IPSS).

MDS with isolated del(5q), as defined in the 2008 WHO classification, is associated with a particular disease phenotype, response to a specific therapy, and favorable prognosis. Mutations in SF3B1, a splicing factor, have been shown to have a strong association with the presence of ring sideroblasts. A complex karyotype, defined as three or more independent cytogenetic abnormalities, is more frequently seen in patients with therapy-related MDS.

The prognostic value of mutations should be interpreted in the context of cytopenias, morphology, proportion of blasts, cytogenetic abnormalities, and co-occurring mutations. Patients with mutations in *DNMT3A,* a methyltransferase, were reported to have worse OS and more rapid evolution to AML [17]. However, mutated SF3B1 co-occurring with DNMT3A mutations may mitigate the negative effect of DNMT3A mutations on survival [18]. Mutations involving *IDH1,* which lead to DNA hypermethylation, were associated with a shorter OS and increased transformation to AML [19]. In a recent analysis of data from 3200 MDS patients, mutations of IDH2 were associated with shorter OS (hazard ratio 1.61, 95% confidence interval [CI] 1.26–2.05; $p = 0.0001$) whereas IDH1 mutations were not significantly associated with OS (HR 1.29, CI: 0.97–1.72; $p = 0.082$).

Table 1.5 Results of NGS-based testing from bone marrow

Gene	Genomic alterations detected	Allele frequency (%)
FLT3	(c.2503G > T; **p.D835Y**)	92%
CCND3	(c.820_826delinsTA; **p.S274***)	40%
DNMT3A	(c.2206C > A; **p.R736S**)	45%
NPM1	(c.860_863dupTCTG; **p.W288Cfs*12**)	N/A
SF3B1	(c.1988C > T; **p.T663I**)	44%
SSBP2-CHD1	Fusion	N/A
WT1	(c.728C > A; **p.S243***)	51%
WT1	(c.707dup; **p.A237Gfs*11**)	39%

The significance of TET2 mutations is not fully established. Although some studies have shown a favorable prognosis [20], a larger study did not identify OS benefit with mono-allelic or bi-allelic TET2 mutations [21]. Driver genes involved in histone modification such as ASXL1 and EZH2 have been shown to be significant predictors of poor OS [21]. *SF3B1* and *SRSF2* are part of the spliceosome and play an important role in RNA splicing. *SF3B1* mutations are present in over 20% of MDS patients and are enriched in myelodysplastic syndrome with ring sideroblasts. Patients with *SF3B1* mutations have a significantly better OS and a reduced incidence of disease progression than patients lacking them [4].

TP53 mutation is associated with a dismal prognosis in all types of MDS, even in the context of allogeneic stem cell transplantation (SCT). *TP53* mutation has been shown to be more predictive of OS than IPSS score [22]. In a study of patients who underwent stem cell transplantation for MDS, mutations in *TP53* (HR, 4.22; P 0.001) and TET2 (HR, 1.68; P = 0.037) were each independently associated with shorter OS [23].

1.8 Case 2: 52-Year-Old Male with Pancytopenia

A 52-year-old male with no significant past medical history presented with chest pain, fatigue, and shortness of breath. Routine blood count detected pancytopenia. A bone marrow biopsy demonstrated a hypercellular marrow with 90% cellularity, dysplastic myelopoiesis and megakaryopoiesis, and increased blasts (25%). Reticulin fibrosis was increased (MF grade 3/3). Blasts were positive for CD34, CD13, CD38, CD117, and CD7. Classical cytogenetic studies revealed a normal male karyotype. Targeted sequencing studies were performed using a NGS-based panel. The results are shown in Table 1.5.

This case would be classified as AML with myelodysplasia-related changes under WHO classification. The patient underwent induction with CPX351 (liposomal daunorubicin + cytarabine) but was refractory to therapy. After reinduction therapy with mitoxantrone, etoposide, and cytarabine, a subsequent bone marrow biopsy showed hypocellular marrow with 5% residual blasts and dyspoietic changes consistent with residual disease. The patient subsequently developed progressive disease with increasing circulating blasts and was started on decitabine and venetoclax.

1.9   Discussion

This case highlights the clinical application of genomic characterization for prognostication of AML. The molecular alterations in AML have been extensively characterized in multiple studies and will be described first. The interpretation of molecular results, classification of prognostic risk groups based on these alterations and methods for minimal/measurable residual disease (MRD) detection will be discussed briefly.

1.9.1   Genetic Alterations in AML

Next generation sequencing studies have expanded our knowledge of the molecular alterations in AML [24–26]. The major functional categories of genes involved in the pathogenesis of AML overlap significantly with the driver genes in MDS (Table 1.3). Grimwade et al. [25] segregated AML into a number of biologically and prognostically distinct subgroups based on patterns of mutual exclusivity between cytogenetic and molecular features (Fig. 1.2). Approximately one-third of AML cases are characterized by the presence of balanced chromosomal rearrangements which are mutually exclusive of mutations in NPM1 and bi-allelic CEBPA. Cases with NPM1 or bi-allelic CEBPA mutations are now separate categories in the WHO classification and account for another third of cases. Complex karyotype/monosomal karyotype/TP53 mutations defines a group with poor prognosis (10% of all cases). TP53 mutations are seen in 45% and complex karyotype in 75% in this group. The remaining cases include those with chromatin/spliceosome mutations, IDH2 mutations, and few cases with no recognized driver mutations. Mutations seen in the various AML subgroups are shown in Fig. 1.3.

1.9.2   ELN Classification Integrating Cytogenetics and Mutation Analysis

The European leukemia network (ELN) genetic risk stratification uses a 3 group classification that incorporates cytogenetic and molecular findings (table 1.6) [27]. Patients with NPM1 mutation and bi-allelic CEBPA mutations are associated with a favorable prognosis in the absence of a high allelic ratio FLT3-ITD mutations (FLT3-ITD [high] is defined as cases that have a > 0.5% ratio of mutant to normal signals), even in the presence of coexisting chromosomal abnormalities [28, 29], However, patients with wild-type NPM1 and FLT3-ITD [high] are associated with a

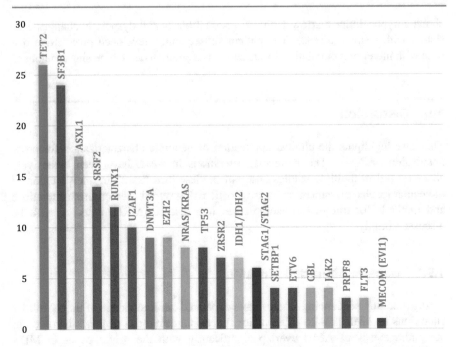

Fig. 1.2 Frequency distribution of the common mutations detected in myelodysplastic syndrome by next generation sequencing. TET2, SF3B1, and ASXL1 are the genes most commonly mutated. The different pathways affected are indicated in different colors. Blue—DNA methylation; Brown—RNA splicing; orange-chromatin modification; sky-blue-signal transduction; Red-others

poor prognosis whereas the combination of mutated NPM1 and FLT3-ITD [high] confers an intermediate prognosis. Other changes in the 2017 ELN classification include addition of mutations in RUNX1, ASXL1, and TP53 in the adverse prognosis group, but not IDH1/2. Monosomal karyotype is defined by the presence of one single monosomy (excluding the sex chromosomes) in association with at least one additional monosomy or structural chromosomal abnormality but excludes core-binding factor AML. A complex karyotype, defined as 3 or more unrelated chromosomal abnormalities in the absence of any of the WHO-designated chromosomal rearrangements, is also associated with an adverse prognosis.

1.9.3   Interpretation of NGS Mutation Panel Results

The implications of the genomic alterations seen in this patient are discussed below in the context of gene function and the effects on protein structure and function.

A stop-gain alteration at codon 274 of the CCND3 gene was detected. The CCND3 gene encodes cyclin D3, which is a critical regulator of cell cycle progression. Mutations of CCND3 have been found in a variety of hematologic

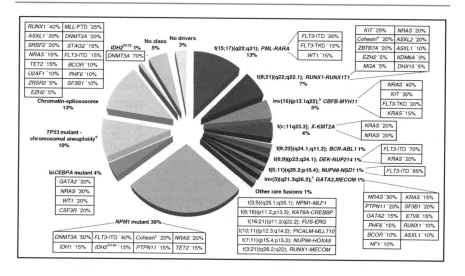

Fig. 1.3 Molecular classes of AML and concurrent gene mutations in adult patients up to the age of ~65 years. The common co-occurring mutations associated with each category are shown in the respective boxes. Data on the frequency of genetic lesions are compiled from the databases of the British Medical Research Council (MRC), the German-Austrian AML Study Group (AMLSG), and from selected studies. (Adapted from Grimwade et al. [25])

malignancies, including acute myeloid leukemia (AML) [30], but the p.S274* mutation detected in this specimen has never been reported, to our knowledge. However, stop-gain mutations lead to premature truncation and loss of function of the protein.

A missense alteration at codon 736 of the DNMT3A gene was detected. The DNMT3A gene encodes a de novo DNA methyltransferase essential for establishing methylation. Somatic mutations in DNMT3A are found in ~30% of normal karyotype AML cases. To our knowledge, the p.R736S mutation detected in this specimen has not been previously reported. However, different changes at the same codon have been frequently reported in hematologic malignancies. Therefore, the p.R736S mutation is expected to be likely pathogenic.

FLT3: A missense alteration at codon 835 of the FLT3 gene was detected. Activating mutations in FLT3 occur commonly in AML, including internal tandem duplication (ITD) and point mutations in the tyrosine kinase domain (TKD), typically at the activation loop residue D835. TKD alterations may be associated with resistance to the FLT3 TKIs (tyrosine kinase inhibitors).

NPM1: A 4-bp insertion of the NPM1 gene was detected. The NPM1 gene encodes nucleophosmin which is involved in ribosomal protein assembly and transport. NPM1 mutations represent frequent genetic alterations in patients with

Table 1.6 Prognostic risk categorization based on cytogenetic and molecular abnormalities

Risk category*	Genetic abnormality
Favorable	t(8;21)(q22;q22.1); *RUNX1-RUNX1T1*
	inv(16)(p13.1q22) or t(16;16)(p13.1;q22); *CBFB-MYH11*
	Mutated *NPM1* without *FLT3*-ITD or with *FLT3*-ITD^{low}
	Bi-allelic mutated *CEBPA*
Intermediate	Mutated *NPM1* and *FLT3*-ITD^{high}†
	Wild-type *NPM1* without *FLT3*-ITD or with *FLT3*-ITD^{low}† (without adverse-risk genetic lesions)
	t(9;11)(p21.3;q23.3); *MLLT3-KMT2A*‡
	Cytogenetic abnormalities not classified as favorable or adverse
Adverse	t(6;9)(p23;q34.1); *DEK-NUP214*
	t(v;11q23.3); *KMT2A* rearranged
	t(9;22)(q34.1;q11.2); *BCR-ABL1*
	inv(3)(q21.3q26.2) or t(3;3)(q21.3;q26.2); *GATA2,MECOM(EVI1)*
	− 5 or del(5q); − 7; − 17/abn(17p)
	Complex karyotype,§ monosomal karyotype‖
	Wild-type *NPM1* and *FLT3*-ITD^{high}†
	Mutated *RUNX1*¶
	Mutated *ASXL1*¶
	Mutated *TP53*#

†Low, low allelic ratio (< 0.5); high, high allelic ratio (> 0.5) by semiquantitative assessment of FLT3-ITD allelic ratio

‡The presence of t(9;11)(p21.3;q23.3) takes precedence over rare, concurrent adverse-risk gene mutations.

§Three or more unrelated chromosome abnormalities in the absence of 1 of the WHO-designated recurring translocations or inversions, that is, t(8;21), inv(16) or t(16;16), t(9;11), t(v;11)(v;q23.3), t(6;9), inv(3) or t(3;3); AML with BCR-ABL1.

‖Defined by the presence of 1 single monosomy (excluding loss of X or Y) in association with at least 1 additional monosomy or structural chromosome abnormality (excluding core-binding factor AML).

¶These markers should not be used as an adverse prognostic marker if they co-occur with favorable-risk AML subtypes.

TP53 mutations are significantly associated with AML with complex and monosomal karyotype Adapted from Dohner H et al. Blood 2017; 129: 424–47.

AML associated with a favorable prognosis [31]. Mutations in the NPM1 gene have been described in approximately 50–60% of AML patients with normal karyotype. The 4-bp insertion in exon 12 of the gene NPM1 is found in 20–30% of AML cases.

SF3B1: A missense alteration at codon 663 of the SF3B1 gene was detected. The SF3B1 gene encodes subunit 1 of the splicing factor 3b, which is important for anchoring the spliceosome to precursor mRNA. SF3B1 mutations are generally associated with favorable outcomes[32]. The p.T663I mutation detected in this specimen has been previously reported in both myeloid and lymphoid malignancies.

SSBP2-CHD1: A rearrangement involving the CHD1 gene on chr 5q15 and SSBP2 gene was detected in this specimen. The CHD1 gene encodes a chromatin-remodeling enzyme that belongs to the chromodomain family of proteins that play an important role in transcriptional regulation and developmental processes. It has been reported that CHD1 is involved in the assembly, shifting, and removal of nucleosomes from the DNA double helix to keep them in an open and transcriptionally active state. Recent reports have shown that CHD1 plays a tumor-suppressor role in prostate cancer and transcriptome sequencing identified CHD1 as a novel partner gene of RUNX1 in acute myeloid leukemia [33]. The SSBP2 gene at 5q14 is suggested to be involved in the DNA damage response and maintenance of genome stability. SSBP2 has recently been identified as a new JAK2 fusion partner in a patient with pre-B cell acute lymphoblastic leukemia [34]. The SSBP2-CHD1 fusion detected is a rare alteration which has been reported once in the literature in an acute undifferentiated leukemia and once in a Ph-like ALL. The clinical significance of this fusion in AML has not been established.

WT1: Two alterations including a nonsense alteration at codon 243 and a frameshift mutation at codon 237 of the WT1 gene were detected. The WT1 gene encodes a zinc finger transcription factor and is involved in tumor-suppressor and oncogenic functions. WT1 mutations are found in 15% of AML cases and are associated with a poor response to chemotherapy [35]. To our knowledge, the p. S243* and p.A237Gfs*11 alterations detected in this specimen have never been reported. However, frameshift and nonsense mutations could lead to premature truncation of the protein and are expected to have a significant deleterious effect.

This case illustrates the difficulty in accurately determining prognosis using current risk stratification criteria. Although the overall mutation pattern fits with the NPM1 mutant group and in the absence of a FLT3-ITD mutation indicates a favorable prognosis, the contribution of the additional mutations like FLT3-TKD, SF3B1 and WT1 to prognosis remains unclear at this time.

1.9.4 Evaluation of Minimal/Measurable Residual Disease (MRD) in Management of AML

The 2017 ELN recommendations include molecular relapse as a new response criterion (complete remission with/without MRD) [27]. Measurable/minimal residual disease denotes the presence of leukemic blasts down to the level of $1:10^4$ to $1:10^6$ white blood cells [36]. MRD quantification provides an objective measure of disease status which can be used to monitor deep remission, predict outcomes, evaluate therapies and identify impending relapse. Multiparameter flow cytometry (MFC) and real-time quantitative polymerase chain reaction (qPCR) are established techniques for MRD evaluation. Next generation sequencing (NGS) based methods and droplet digital PCR are newer technologies currently in evaluation. European leukemia network MRD recommendations for MFC recommends a comprehensive flow cytometry panel with a combination approach for assessing residual disease—using leukemia-associated immunophenotype (LAIP) as well as different from normal (DfN) strategies [36]. The advantages of the DfN approach, which is based on the identification of aberrant differentiation/maturation profiles at follow-up, include applicability in cases where the diagnostic immunophenotype is not available and cases with immunophenotypic shifts.

There are multiple approaches for molecular MRD assessment. Classical real-time qPCR for recurrent translocations and selected mutations such as NPM1 has high sensitivity (10^{-4} to 10^{-6}) and specificity and is currently considered the gold standard, but is limited to approximately 40% of AML patients. Many other common mutations such as DMMT3A, ASXL1, and TET2 genes may represent clonal hematopoiesis [12], especially in the older population, and should not be used in isolation. In addition, mutations in FLT3-ITD, FLT3-TKD, NRAS, KRAS, IDH1, IDH2, and MLL-PTD are frequently lost or gained in relapse. However, these markers are informative in combination with a second or multiple MRD markers.

Next generation sequencing-based methods have limited sensitivity of approximately 1%. Methods using error-corrected NGS are being tested to increase sensitivity. Droplet digital PCR can be used to detect mutations at levels of 0.1% or lower, but each mutation requires a specific assay to be developed. In the allogenic stem cell transplantation setting, assessment of donor/recipient chimerism in blood or bone marrow using fragment analysis of short tandem repeats is widely used. However, this method lacks sensitivity and is not recommended for MRD detection or monitoring. Monitoring of germline variants in leukemia-associated genes like RUNX1 from the diagnostic sample could also be useful as markers of donor/recipient chimerism in the sample.

1.9.5 Future Perspectives

Large-scale sequencing projects over the last 10 years such as The Cancer genome Atlas (TCGA) project have revolutionized our understanding of the molecular genetics of AML. Although the average AML genome has approximately 15 coding mutations, there are over 200 genes with recurrent mutations. It is now feasible in a clinical setting to characterize the relevant coding genes together with the cytogenetic alterations including translocations and copy number alterations. Multiple studies are ongoing to understand how the various combinations of genomic alterations affect response to therapy and prognosis. The 2017 ELN classification incorporates a few molecular alterations in a prognostic risk classification for clinical implementation. Further revisions are expected as our knowledge expands. Big data initiatives like the HARMONY platform and Beat AML will be critical to reach the statistical power needed for multifactorial analysis.

Combination therapies targeting multiple pathways such as the combination of hypomethylating agents with Bcl-2 inhibitors have shown great promise in the clinic [37, 38] and are active across various genetic subtypes of AML and MDS. Techniques such as single cell sequencing and gene expression profiling will offer insight into the signaling pathways and enable multi-pathway targeting in the future whereby additional targeted agents directed at driver mutations in genes like IDH1/2 and FLT3 can be added to treatment regimens to further improve outcomes. Understanding the role of the tumor microenvironment and the biology of leukemic stem cells are rapidly evolving. Genetic mutations may determine the susceptibility of particular subtypes of myeloid malignancies to various immunotherapeutic approaches as well.

References

1. Vallespi T et al (1998) Diagnosis, classification, and cytogenetics of myelodysplastic syndromes. Haematologica 83(3):258–275
2. Ogawa S (2019) Genetics of MDS. Blood 133(10):1049–1059
3. Desai P, Roboz GJ (2019) Clonal Hematopoiesis and therapy related MDS/AML. Best Pract Res Clin Haematol 32(1):13–23
4. Cazzola M, Della Porta MG, Malcovati L (2013) The genetic basis of myelodysplasia and its clinical relevance. Blood 122(25), 4021–4034
5. Delhommeau F et al (2009) Mutation in TET2 in myeloid cancers. N Engl J Med 360 (22):2289–2301
6. Ley TJ et al (2010) DNMT3A mutations in acute myeloid leukemia. N Engl J Med 363 (25):2424–2433
7. Nikoloski G et al (2010) Somatic mutations of the histone methyltransferase gene EZH2 in myelodysplastic syndromes. Nat Genet 42(8):665–667
8. Papaemmanuil E et al (2011) Somatic SF3B1 mutation in myelodysplasia with ring sideroblasts. N Engl J Med 365(15):1384–1395
9. Beerman I et al (2010) Functionally distinct hematopoietic stem cells modulate hematopoietic lineage potential during aging by a mechanism of clonal expansion. Proc Natl Acad Sci U S A 107(12):5465–5470
10. Welch JS et al (2012) The origin and evolution of mutations in acute myeloid leukemia. Cell 150(2):264–278
11. Jaiswal S et al (2014) Age-related clonal hematopoiesis associated with adverse outcomes. N Engl J Med 371(26):2488–2498
12. Steensma DP et al (2015) Clonal hematopoiesis of indeterminate potential and its distinction from myelodysplastic syndromes. Blood 126(1):9–16
13. Kwok B et al (2015) MDS-associated somatic mutations and clonal hematopoiesis are common in idiopathic cytopenias of undetermined significance. Blood 126(21):2355–2361
14. Kakosaiou K et al (2018) ASXL1 mutations in AML are associated with specific clinical and cytogenetic characteristics. Leuk Lymphoma 59(10):2439–2446
15. Brendel C et al. (2015) Oncogenic NRAS primes primary acute myeloid leukemia cells for differentiation. PLoS One 10(4), e0123181
16. Greif PA et al (2012) RUNX1 mutations in cytogenetically normal acute myeloid leukemia are associated with a poor prognosis and up-regulation of lymphoid genes. Haematologica 97 (12):1909–1915
17. Walter MJ et al (2011) Recurrent DNMT3A mutations in patients with myelodysplastic syndromes. Leukemia 25(7):1153–1158
18. Bejar R et al (2012) Validation of a prognostic model and the impact of mutations in patients with lower-risk myelodysplastic syndromes. J Clin Oncol 30(27):3376–3382
19. Thol F et al (2010) IDH1 mutations in patients with myelodysplastic syndromes are associated with an unfavorable prognosis. Haematologica 95(10):1668–1674
20. Kosmider O et al (2009) TET2 mutation is an independent favorable prognostic factor in myelodysplastic syndromes (MDSs). Blood 114(15):3285–3291

21. Bejar R et al (2011) Clinical effect of point mutations in myelodysplastic syndromes. N Engl J Med 364(26):2496–2506
22. Horiike S et al (2003) Configuration of the TP53 gene as an independent prognostic parameter of myelodysplastic syndrome. Leuk Lymphoma 44(6):915–922
23. Bejar R et al (2014) Somatic mutations predict poor outcome in patients with myelodysplastic syndrome after hematopoietic stem-cell transplantation. J Clin Oncol 32(25):2691–2698
24. Cancer Genome Atlas Research N et al. (2013) Genomic and epigenomic landscapes of adult de novo acute myeloid leukemia. N Engl J Med 368(22), 059–74
25. Grimwade D, Ivey A, Huntly BJ (2016) Molecular landscape of acute myeloid leukemia in younger adults and its clinical relevance. Blood 127(1):29–41
26. Papaemmanuil E et al (2016) Genomic classification and prognosis in acute Myeloid Leukemia. N Engl J Med 374(23):2209–2221
27. Dohner H et al (2017) Diagnosis and management of AML in adults: 2017 ELN recommendations from an international expert panel. Blood 129(4):424–447
28. Micol JB, et al. (2009) The role of cytogenetic abnormalities in acute myeloid leukemia with NPM1 mutations and no FLT3 internal tandem duplication. Blood 114(20), 4601–2; author reply 4602–3
29. Schlenk RF et al (2013) The value of allogeneic and autologous hematopoietic stem cell transplantation in prognostically favorable acute myeloid leukemia with double mutant CEBPA. Blood 122(9):1576–1582
30. Matsuo H et al (2018) Recurrent CCND3 mutations in MLL-rearranged acute myeloid leukemia. Blood Adv 2(21):2879–2889
31. Heath EM et al (2017) Biological and clinical consequences of NPM1 mutations in AML. Leukemia 31(4):798–807
32. Cazzola M et al (2013) Biologic and clinical significance of somatic mutations of SF3B1 in myeloid and lymphoid neoplasms. Blood 121(2):260–269
33. Yao H et al (2015) Transcriptome sequencing reveals CHD1 as a novel fusion partner of RUNX1 in acute myeloid leukemia with t(5;21)(q21;q22). Mol Cancer 14:81
34. Roberts KG et al (2014) Targetable kinase-activating lesions in Ph-like acute lymphoblastic leukemia. N Engl J Med 371(11):1005–1015
35. Paschka P et al (2008) Wilms' tumor 1 gene mutations independently predict poor outcome in adults with cytogenetically normal acute myeloid leukemia: a cancer and leukemia group B study. J Clin Oncol 26(28):4595–4602
36. Schuurhuis GJ et al (2018) Minimal/measurable residual disease in AML: a consensus document from the European LeukemiaNet MRD working party. Blood 131(12):1275–1291
37. Aldoss I et al (2018) Efficacy of the combination of venetoclax and hypomethylating agents in relapsed/refractory acute myeloid leukemia. Haematologica 103(9):e404–e407
38. DiNardo CD et al (2019) Venetoclax combined with decitabine or azacitidine in treatment-naive, elderly patients with acute myeloid leukemia. Blood 133(1):7–17

Genetics and Diagnostic Approach to Lymphoblastic Leukemia/Lymphoma

2

Michelle Afkhami, Feras Ally, Vinod Pullarkat, and Raju K. Pillai

Contents

M. Afkhami (✉) · F. Ally · V. Pullarkat · R. K. Pillai
City of Hope Medical Center, 1500 E Duarte Rd., Duarte, CA 91010, USA
e-mail: mafkhami@coh.org

R. K. Pillai
e-mail: rpillai@coh.org

© Springer Nature Switzerland AG 2021
V. Pullarkat and G. Marcucci (eds.), *Biology and Treatment of Leukemia and Bone Marrow Neoplasms*, Cancer Treatment and Research 181,
https://doi.org/10.1007/978-3-030-78311-2_2

2.1   Introduction

B- and T-cell lymphoblastic leukemia/lymphoma (commonly termed acute lymphoblastic leukemia [B-ALL/T-ALL]) are clonal neoplasms of lymphoid progenitors. Lymphoblastic leukemia/lymphoma is the most common childhood malignancy, which also occurs in adults with a lower incidence rate. These neoplasms are characterized by arrest of maturation and rapid proliferation of the early precursor hematopoietic cells called blasts which accumulate in bone marrow, peripheral blood, and other tissues. It is denoted lymphoblastic lymphoma (LBL) when it primarily involves an extramedullary site with minimal or no blood or bone marrow involvement. Acute lymphoblastic leukemia has been reported to have higher incidence in Hispanics [1–3].

Involvement of lymph nodes or extranodal sites such as liver, spleen, or central nervous system (CNS) is frequent in B-lymphoblastic lymphoma (B-LBL), whereas it is the most common presentation for T-lymphoblastic lymphoma (T-LBL). B- and T-ALL/LBL harbor a wide variety of distinct genetic alterations, including recurrent chromosomal changes, fusions, mutations, expression, and copy number variations affecting multiple signaling pathways. These genomic alterations are used for diagnosis, prognosis, and therapy selection.

A breakthrough in the understanding of ALL genetics was the discovery of t(9;22) (q34;q11.2) (Philadelphia chromosome) resulting in *BCR-ABL1* fusion, in a discrete subset of B-ALL cases. This subtype of ALL has distinct prognosis and treatment includes targeted therapy with tyrosine kinase inhibitors. Based on genetic findings, two main categories for B-ALL/LBL have been introduced in the current WHO classification: B-ALL/LBL with recurrent genetic abnormalities and B-ALL/LBL not otherwise specified. Many of the genetic abnormalities involved can be detected by conventional cytogenetics, but some are difficult to detect by regular cytogenetic analysis and might need other techniques such as next-generation sequencing (NGS). In this chapter we will briefly review all the genomic subtypes of B- and T-ALL/LBL, then will discuss morphology, immunophenotype, genomics, and molecular techniques used to approach diagnosis, prognosis, and treatment in the context of three illustrative cases.

2.2 B-lymphoblastic Leukemia/Lymphoma

2.2.1 Epidemiology and Risk Factors

B-Acute lymphoblastic leukemia/lymphoblastic lymphoma (B-ALL/LBL) is the most common childhood hematologic malignancy constituting about 25% of all cancers diagnosed in children aged 0–14 years old and 80% of all childhood leukemia cases. This is also common in adolescents and young adults with less favorable prognosis. In adults, ALL is also considered a rare disease and accounts for 20% of all adult leukemia cases [2, 5].

The risk of developing ALL is highest in children younger than 5 years of age. The risk then declines slowly until the mid-20 s and begins to rise again after age 50 [1, 4]. The prognosis for childhood B-ALL has improved remarkably over the last 4 decades due to optimization of chemotherapy regimens and better understanding of the genetics of this disease, resulting in long-term disease-free survival in >90% of patients. By contrast, long-term disease-free survival in adults is achieved in around 40% of cases and the 5-year survival rate for people age 20 and older is 35% and for age under 20 is about 90% [6, 7]. This difference might be due to both disease-related factors such as higher frequency of unfavorable genomic abnormalities in adults, as well as patient-related factors, such as decreased tolerance to chemotherapy due to other comorbidities in older adults.

Some genetic and environmental factors that predispose to ALL have been reported. These include certain risk factors such as age, race/ethnicity (more common in Whites than African Americans), gender (slight male predominance) radiation exposure, chemical exposure including benzene or chemotherapy, specific viruses, certain genetic syndromes such as Down, Klinefelter, Bloom, and Li-Fraumeni syndromes, Fanconi anemia, ataxia-telangiectasia, and neurofibromatosis [8–12]. Higher incidence of Ph-like subset has been reported in Hispanics related to inherited *GATA3* variant [2, 8].

Acute leukemia can be de novo or therapy-related. Therapy-related ALL resulting from exposure to cytotoxic chemotherapy/radiation accounts for 10–15% of all therapy-related leukemia [13].

2.2.2 Genomic Classification of B-Lymphoblastic Leukemia

B-lymphoblastic leukemia/lymphoma is a heterogeneous disease with a wide variety of chromosomal abnormalities and genetic alterations. Approximately 75% of cases will have recurrent chromosomal changes detected by conventional cytogenetics including hyperdiploidy, hypodiploidy, translocations, and chromosomal deletion or amplifications [14].

The 2016 World Health Organization (WHO) classification of tumors of the hematopoietic and lymphoid tissues currently classifies the precursor B-lymphoid neoplasms to B-lymphoblastic leukemia/lymphoma with recurrent genetic

Table 2.1 WHO 2016 classification of B-ALL	B-lymphoblastic leukemia/lymphoma with recurrent genetic abnormalities
	• Hypodiploidy
	• Hyperdiploidy
	• *BCR-ABL1*, t(9;22)(q34;q11.2)
	• *KMT2A (MLL)* rearranged, t(v;11q23)
	• *ETV6-RUNX1*, t(12;21)(p13;q22)
	• *TCF3-PBX1*, t(1;19)(q23;p13.3)
	• *IL3-IGH*, t(5;14)(q31;q32)
	• iAMP21, intrachromosomal amplification of chromosome 21
	• *BCR-ABL1*-like or Ph-like, translocations involving tyrosine kinases (TKs) or cytokine receptors
	B-lymphoblastic leukemia/lymphoma, not otherwise specified

abnormalities and B-lymphoblastic leukemia/lymphoma not otherwise specified (NOS) [1, 15–21]. The specific recurrent genetic abnormalities are listed in Table 2.1.

2.3 B-ALL with Recurrent Genetic Abnormalities

2.3.1 B-ALL with BCR/ABL1

One of the more frequent cytogenetic alterations in adult B-cell acute lymphoblastic leukemia is *BCR-ABL1* fusion resulting from t(9;22)(q34;q11.2) translocation, also known as the Philadelphia (Ph) chromosome. This genetic abnormality occurs in about 25% of adult cases and about 5% of childhood B-ALL cases. Rearrangement involving the major breakpoint in the BCR gene results in a 210-kD protein, which is detected in half of the adult cases and less commonly in pediatric ALL [1]. The minor breakpoint encodes a 190-kDa protein is more prevalent in both adult and pediatric cases occurring in 50 and 90% of cases, respectively. The translocation results in a constitutively active *ABL1* kinase. Multiple downstream signaling pathways are activated due to this oncogenic fusion. including RAS/MEK/ERK (activation of transcription factors, including NF-kB), PI-3 kinase/AKT (cell growth, cell survival, and inhibition of apoptosis), and JAK-STAT (cell growth and survival) pathways [16–18]. This subtype has been reported to have the more immature cell of origin compared to other B-ALL [19].

2.3.2 B-ALL with KMT2A (MLL) Rearrangement

Rearrangement of *KMT2A* gene on chromosome11 t(v;11q23.3) with a variety of fusion partners is a recurrent cytogenetic abnormality that is most common in infants with B-ALL in whom it carries a particularly poor prognosis. KMT2A rearrangement constitutes about 10% of adult B-ALL and is associated with exposure to topoisomerase II inhibitors, in which case it is associated with a short latency period. This rearrangement is most commonly detected by conventional cytogenetics or by fluorescence in situ hybridization using a KMT2A break apart probe. Most commonly occurring as t(4;11) resulting in *KMT2A-AFF1* (MLL-AF4) fusion, these blasts usually have a pro-B immunophenotype, with expression of CD19 and CD15 and lack of expression of CD10 and CD24. In general, *KMT2A* rearrangement carries a poor prognosis and outcome is particularly poor in infantile B-ALL [20–22].

2.3.3 ETV6/RUNX1 t(12;21)

The translocation t(12;21)(p13.2;q22.1) leading to *ETV6-RUNX1* (TEL/AML1) fusion is present in about 25% of childhood ALL where it is associated with an excellent prognosis. This abnormality however is present in only less than 5% of adult ALL. This is a cryptic translocation not detectable by conventional cytogenetics and requires FISH study for its diagnosis [23, 24].

2.3.4 *TCF3/PBX1* t(1;19)

This subset of B-ALL harbors a fusion between *TCF3* (also known as E2A) gene on chromosome 19 and *PBX1* gene on chromosome 1. It comprises about 6% of childhood B-ALL and is less common in adults. This subtype does not appear to have prognostic relevance. Blasts typically express CD9 and lack CD34 expression on immunophenotyping [25, 26].

2.3.5 Hyperdiploidy

Leukemic blasts in this subtype carry more than 50 chromosomes (usually <66). It is seen in about 25% of children but is not common in adults [20, 21]. Extra copies of chromosomes 4,14,21, and X are the most common and structural abnormalities are uncommon. These cases have an immunophenotype typical of B-ALL. In cases of hyperdiploid ALL, one would expect that most of the genes involved are located on chromosomes with extra copies, e.g., chromosomes 4, 6, 10, 14, 17, 18, 21, and X. However, overexpression of *SH3BP5 (located on 3p24)* and *CREBBP* (located on 16p13.3) genes has been reported. The prognosis of hyperdiploid B-ALL is very favorable with a cure rate in >90% of children [27–29].

2.3.6 Hypodiploidy

Hypodiploid B-ALL blasts by definition contain less than 46 chromosomes. This subtype occurs in about 5% of B-ALL in both children and adults. Hypodiploid ALL has been further divided into subtypes based on the chromosome number. The low-hypodiploid subtype (defined as 33–39 chromosomes) carries *TP53* mutations in more than 90% of cases, and the majority also show monosomy 17 by cytogenetic studies. In addition, in about 50% of cases they harbor lymphoid transcription factor IKZF2 deletions, or mutations in *CDKN2A*, *CDKN2B*, and *RB1*. The near-haploid ALL with 23–29 chromosomes often have *RAS* mutations, IKZF3 deletions, or receptor tyrosine kinase alterations. The other subtypes are high hypodiploid ALL with 40–43 chromosomes and near-diploid ALLs with 44–45 chromosomes, with the latter having a better prognosis than other subtypes. Hypodiploidy can be missed by conventional cytogenetics in some cases if the low-hypodiploid or near-haploid clone has undergone endoduplication resulting in increased chromosome number and should be suspected in cases of chromosome number discrepancy between FISH and cytogenetic studies [29–31].

2.3.7 IL3/IGH, t(5;14)

The t(5;14)(q31.1;q32.1), which juxtaposes the interleukin-3 (IL3) gene on chromosome 5 with the immunoglobulin heavy-chain (IGH) gene on chromosome 14 has similar immunophenotype as other B-ALL. This subtype usually has circulating eosinophilia which is not part of the malignant clone. This peripheral eosinophilia can cause symptoms related to release of toxic granules such as cardiac disease [1, 32].

2.3.8 Intrachromosomal Amplification of Chromosome 21 (iAMP21)

More common in children, this is a rare subtype detected by FISH with probe for *RUNX1* or on NGS analysis, which shows the amplification of a portion of chromosome 21. Interestingly the *RUNX1* gene itself does not appear to be involved in leukemogenesis and other amplified genes are probably the contributing factor. It is considered an adverse prognostic factor in children [1, 33, 34].

2.3.9 Ph-Like ALL

The use of genomic technologies has led to the discovery of a new subgroup of B-ALL in 2009; lacking *BCR-ABL1* rearrangement (t9;22), but harboring a kinase-activated gene expression profile similar to Ph-positive ALL. This entity is called Philadelphia chromosome-like (Ph-like) or *BCR-ABL1* like ALL and is associated with an unfavorable outcome. This Ph-like subgroup is extremely heterogeneous with regard to genomic alterations and is difficult to diagnose without complex molecular testing [35, 36]. Ph-like ALL is currently included under the category of ALL with recurrent genetic abnormalities. It is characterized by a distinct gene expression profile, chromosomal rearrangements, and both copy number alterations (CNAs) and sequence alterations that affect lymphoid development, tumor suppressor, cytokine receptor, kinase, and other signaling pathways. This subtype has constitutive activation of signal transduction pathways, often due to tyrosine kinase fusions other than *BCR-ABL1*. Ph-like ALL comprises 20–25% of B-ALL in adolescents and young adults and is associated with worse relapse and survival rates, however, the frequency and biology of this in older populations (>65) is not clearly known [37–40]. *GATA3* germline alterations may explain the increased incidence of Ph-like ALL in Hispanics and native Americans relative to Europeans and may underlie their poorer outcomes [2, 3, 8, 41]. Age-related differences may be due to disease-related factors such as a higher frequency of unfavorable genomic abnormalities in adults, and patient-related factors including decreased tolerance to chemotherapy for other medical conditions; however, this needs to be better defined with more precise risk criteria.

There are two main subgroups of Ph-like B-lymphoblastic leukemia. The first group is marked by overexpression of cytokine receptor-like factor 2 (*CRLF2*), which is seen in around 50% of cases of Ph-like B-ALL [35–43]. Often this overexpression is driven by fusions involving the *CRLF2* gene, including *P2RY8-CRLF2* and *IGH-CRLF2* fusions [44–53]. About half of these *CRLF2*-rearranged cases also carry *JAK* mutations, with *JAK2* R683G mutation being the most common. This mutation results in *JAK-STAT* pathway activation and could be amenable to therapies involving *JAK* inhibition. The second major subgroup of Ph-like cases has fusions that involve other tyrosine kinases, including *JAK2, ABL1, ABL2, CSF1R*, and *PDGFRB* or rearrangements causing truncation and activation of EPOR. Fusions affecting kinases such as *ABL1, ABL2, CSF1R*, and *PDGFRB* could potentially be targeted with *ABL*-type tyrosine kinase inhibitors, whereas those affecting the *JAK-STAT* pathway (including EPOR) could respond to *JAK* inhibitors [54–60].

2.4 B-ALL Not-Otherwise Specified

This subtype has the classic morphologic and immunophenotypic characteristics of other B-ALL. However, they do not have the genetic abnormalities with known prognostic impact. These abnormalities including *PAX5, RAS, TP53, PTPN11,* and *IKZF1* mutations which can be seen in all subtypes of ALL. *PTPN11* gene encodes the protein tyrosine phosphatase SHP-2, which is involved in the regulation of the RAS/MAPK pathway. Some abnormalities such as del(6q), del(9p), and del(12p) are not specific for ALL and some such as *TCF3/HLF* rearrangements are specific, but very rare and hence not included under ALL with recurrent genetic abnormalities [61–63].

2.4.1   *TCF3* (E2A)/HLF, t(17;19)

These lymphoid blasts harbor a translocation between *TCF3* (also known as *E2A*) gene on chromosome 19 and *HLF* (hepatic leukemia factor) on chromosome 17. B-ALL with translocation t(17;19)(q22;p13) has been reported to be associated with hypercalcemia, disseminated intravascular coagulation, and a normal karyotype. Although very rare the t(17;19)(q22;p13) can be detected by FISH analysis. The fusion *E2A-HLF* transcript was amplified by RT-PCR and sequenced and revealed a type I rearrangement with a long insertion (146 nucleotides) between *E2A* exon 13 and HLF exon 4. E2A/HLF fusion was described in an ALL patient with disseminated intravascular coagulation and a normal karyotype [25, 64].

2.4.2   *IKZF1* Alterations

Rearrangements of the *IKZF1* gene have been observed in both lymphoid and myeloid malignancies. Sequence mutations and deletions of the *IKZF1* gene, which encodes the lymphoid transcription factor IKAROS, occur frequently in Philadelphia-positive (Ph+) acute lymphoblastic leukemia (ALL) and has been associated with poor outcome. The *IKZF1* deletion is also associated with Ph-like ALL [65–75].

2.5   T-lymphoblastic Leukemia/lymphoma

Precursor T-lymphoblastic leukemia/lymphoma or T acute lymphoblastic leukemia/lymphoma (T- ALL/LBL) is characterized by blasts of small to medium-size involving blood or/and bone marrow (leukemic presentation) or infiltration of thymus (mediastinal) or nodal or extranodal sites such as skin, tonsils, spleen, liver, testicle, and CNS (lymphoma presentation). When extramedullary tissue is primarily involved, the peripheral blood might have circulating lymphoblasts. However, the bone marrow blasts should be more than 25% if a diagnosis of leukemia is to be made. The previous classification of pro- and pre-T-ALL is now encompassed under the early T precursor leukemia (ETP-ALL) subtype accounting for 10–13% of childhood and 5–10% of adult T-ALL.

Prognosis and predictive factors

T-ALL in childhood is a higher risk disease than B-ALL, and associated with a higher risk of induction failure, early relapse, and isolated CNS relapse [76]. Minimal residual disease following therapy is a strong adverse prognostic factor [77, 78]. In adult protocols, T-ALL is treated similarly to other types of ALL. The prognosis of T-LBL, like that of other lymphomas, depends on patient age, disease stage, and lactate dehydrogenase levels [79]. Although controversial, most recent data supports the fact that T-ALL and ETP-ALL have similar outcomes [80–82].

Immunophenotype

The T-lymphoblasts usually express TdT, CD1a (heterogeneous), CD2, cytoplasmic and membranous CD3, CD4, CD5, CD7, and CD8. Of these markers, only CD3 is considered lineage specific. Co-expression of CD4 and CD8, TAL1, and CD10 positivity can occasionally be seen [1, 83]. TAL1 expression does not correlate with the presence of *TAL1* gene alteration [84, 85]. Aberrant expression of CD79a (10%), CD13, and CD33 (19–32%) can be seen in some cases [86–88]. Association of activating mutations of FLT3 with KIT expression has been also reported [89, 90]. Occurrence of myeloid markers per se does not indicate ambiguous lineage.

ETP-ALL expresses CD7 without expression of CD5, CD8, and CD1a. It can show myeloid markers expression including CD13, CD33, CD34, KIT (CD117), HLA-DR, CD11b, and CD65. Blasts also express cytoplasmic or rarely surface CD3 and in some cases CD2 and/or CD4 [1].

Genomic alterations in T-ALL/LBL

One of the most common genetic alterations in T-ALL occurs in *NOTCH1* gene, which encodes a protein critical for early T-cell development. Activating *NOTCH1* mutations are reported in 50% of cases and involve the extracellular heterodimerization domain or the C-terminal PEST domain of *NOTCH1*. Increased *NOTCH1* signaling leads to *MYC* activation, which is a downstream target of *NOTCH1* gene. Mutation is the MTOR pathway gene *FBXW7* has been seen in 30% of cases, which is normally a negative regulator of *NOTCH1* and these mutations increase the half-life of the *NOTCH1* protein [91–94]. Somatic *TP53* mutations are found in 16% ALL and are associated with adverse outcomes and found to be more frequent in T-ALL than in B-ALL. These inactivate the tumor suppressor p53 protein that plays a crucial role in cell cycle regulation and apoptosis after DNA damage [27, 30].

Mutations of the *PHF6* gene have mostly been reported in male patients with T-ALL. The *PHF6* gene on the X chromosome encodes a plant homeodomain (PHD) protein containing four nuclear localization signals and two imperfect PHD zinc finger domains with a proposed role in transcriptional regulation and/or chromatin remodeling [95–103]. *JAK1* mutations are more prevalent among adult and childhood subjects with T-ALL compared to B-ALL and these are associated with poor prognosis and a high risk of treatment failure [104–108].

The molecular signature of ETP-ALL is similar to normal early thymocyte precursors and is different from other T-ALL subtypes. Overexpression of CD34, *KIT, GATA2, CD44, and CEBPA* has been reported. Mutations in myeloid-related genes such as *FLT3, KRAS, NRAS*, and *DNMT3A* are more commonly reported in this entity [109–113].

Cytogenetic aberrations occur in about 50–70% of T-ALL/LBL [1]. These often involve rearrangements of the T-cell receptor (TCR) alpha and delta genes followed by TCR beta and gamma abnormalities [114, 115]. However, simultaneous presence of IGH gene rearrangements is found in up to 20% of cases [116, 117]. Most common genes involved are transcription factors *TLX1* (also called *HOX11*) at 10q24 (7% of childhood and 30% of adult cases) and *TLX3* (20% of childhood and 10–15% of adult cases) [114]. Rearrangements in other genes are found including *KMT2A* (*MLL*), *MYC*, *TCF3*, *TAL1*, *STIL*, *PICALM*, *MLLT10*, *NUP98*, *LCK*, *LMO*, *LYL1*, *RBTN1*, and *RBTN2* [114, 118–120]. The *TLX1* gene alterations have been reported to have a favorable prognosis [121]. The fusion of *PICALM-MLLT10* (also known as *CALM-AF10*) resulting from the t(10;11)(p12;q14) is one of the known recurrent fusions in T-ALL but is also reported in AML and mixed-lineage leukemia. The prognosis for patients with *PICALM-MLLT10* fusion may vary depending on the immunophenotype and the presence of *EZH2* mutations [122–128].

NUP214-ABL1 fusion resulting in a constitutively activated tyrosine kinase have been found in T-ALL and Ph-like ALL and may be targetable by tyrosine kinase inhibitors [129–134]. Next-generation sequencing (NGS) studies are often required to identify gene fusions in T-ALL, since in many cases, these rearrangements are not detected by conventional karyotyping.

2.6 Diagnostic Work up of ALL

The national comprehensive cancer network (NCCN) guidelines for acute lymphoblastic leukemia recommends molecular characterization of ALL to include analysis of G-Banded metaphase chromosomes, FISH studies for the major recurrent genetic abnormalities, and RT-PCR for *BCR-ABL1* (p190 and p210). Furthermore, additional testing is encouraged for gene fusions and other mutations if a case is found to be *BCR-ABL1* negative. Additional optional tests include array comparative genomic hybridization in cases of aneuploidy or failed karyotyping [135].

FISH studies are more readily available in most laboratories and are highly specific for selected rearrangements such as those involving IGH. However, this method may not be practical for general screening in ALL cases due to the broad variety of rearrangements that can be present. To expedite a diagnosis and facilitate most appropriate therapy for the patient, RNA sequencing represents the most optimal option if available.

Many laboratories now have NGS assays for acute leukemia ranging from targeted genes starting from 20 genes to whole exome sequencing. These assays are mainly designed to detect mutations and fusions using PCR, Sanger sequencing, RT-PCR, and next-generation sequencing methods. Gene expression assays are not widely available in clinical laboratories.

Identification of Ph-like ALL remains the most challenging issue for initial work up of B-ALL and is critical for its prognostication. Many of the reported strategies are not widely available in clinical practice. Roberts et al. have used an 8-gene TaqMan low-density array (LDA) by PCR for definitive identification of Ph-Like ALL. In cases with high *CRLF* expression the *CRLF2* rearrangement status was assessed with FISH analysis and *JAK1, JAK2* mutations status by Sanger sequencing. The remaining cases with low expression of *CRLF2* were tested with an RT-PCR assay for 41 known kinase fusions transcripts. If these cases had no kinase fusions, then whole transcriptome sequencing was done [136].

Chiaretti et al. recently summarized the testing strategies that different groups have taken to identify Ph-like cases [137]. These assays include an assorted combination of various methods including FISH, LDA, RT-PCR, NGS (RNAseq, Whole exome sequencing, Whole genome sequencing) (17,20), or more simplified approaches including RT-PCR for known fusion transcripts, *JAK2* mutations, and *CRLF2* rearrangement [38, 41].

A stepwise testing strategy starting with an initial LDA assay to determine if the leukemia is pH-like would be more cost effective. However, if the case is determined to be Ph-like, additional testing will be required in a reflex manner, which can be time consuming and might have the risk of having insufficient tissue for further sequential analysis. Diagnosis of Ph-like ALL remains a challenge, particularly in resource poor settings.

2.7 Our Approach to Genomic Testing of ALL

At our facility, the majority of B-ALL cases seen are in adults and we perform a combination of cytogenetics, FISH, RT-PCR, DNAseq, RNAseq, and NGS studies on all initial and relapsed B-ALL cases. These assays were designed with consideration of the frequency of the alterations found in the population seen at our cancer center, which is enriched for Ph-like cases given the large Latino population we servevp.

The use of NGS allows for the detection of gene mutations and fusions that involve a targeted partner. This means that novel fusions can also be detected as long as one of the affected genes is included in the panel. Our testing strategy is depicted in Fig. 2.1. The genes tested in our NGS mutation and fusion panel are shown in Table 2.2.

Our RNAseq assay was designed to assess previously described as well as novel kinase gene fusions in ALL. However, we found that FISH studies for IGH rearrangement were also necessary as *IGH-CRLF2* or *IGH-EPOR* translocations in the case of Ph-like ALL could be missed in cases of rearrangement involving regions outside of primers used. To increase the odds of detection, especially for cases with potential *JAK1* and *JAK2* mutations, we evaluate the CRLF2 expression level by RNAseq and reflex to FISH IGH testing in cases with high expression.

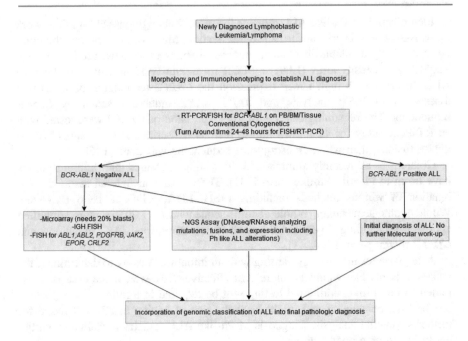

Fig. 2.1 City of Hope testing algorithm for initial work up of B-ALL

There are multiple advantages of doing comprehensive genomic testing upfront for ALL patients using our methodology. These include a faster turnaround time assay as a majority of the relevant alterations are included in one assay. Such a strategy would be cost effective in the long term and detect most Ph-like ALL cases when initially screened by exclusion of Ph-positive ALL by FISH/PCR.

The genomic heterogeneity of Ph-like ALL is broad, and although many of the findings have relevance across age groups; additional research is still necessary to understand implications of particular findings for therapy in different age groups, for instance, response to immune-based treatments and outcomes of allogeneic hematopoietic stem cell transplantation. Understanding the evolution of disease with comparison between the initial and relapsed clones might help with the development of customized minimal residual disease assays and further optimize treatment for this poor prognostic subtype [138–142].

Some illustrative cases evaluated using our diagnostic strategy are described below.

Table 2.2 Hematologic malignancy mutation assay: entire coding region mutation analysis of 135 genes

BL1	ARID1A	ASXL1	ATM	B2M	BCL2	BCL6
BCOR	BCORL1	BIRC3	BRAF	BTK	CALR	CARD11
CBL	CBL-B	CCND1	CCND3	CD38	CD3E	CD3G
CD79A	CD79B	CDK4	CDK7	CDKN1B	CDKN2A	CDKN2B
CDKN2C	CEBPA	CHD2	CRBN	CREBBP	CSF3R	CUX1
CXCR4	DDx3x	DIS3	DNMT3A	E2F1	EGFR	EP300
ETV6	EZH2	FBXW7	FGFR3	FH	FLT3	FAM46C
FOXO1	GATA1	GATA2	GNA13	GNAS	HCK	HRAS
ID3	IDH1	IDH2	IGLL5	*IKZF1*	IL6	IL7R
	IRF4	JAK1	JAK2	JAK3	KDM6A	KIT
KMT2A	KMT2C	KMT2D	KRAS	LCK	LMO2	MAPK1
MEF2B	MGA	MIR 142	MPL	MYC	MYD88	NFKB2
NOTCH1	NOTCH2	NPM1	NRAS	NTRK1	PAX5	PDCD1
PDGFRA	PHF6	PIGA	PIK3CA	PIK3CD	PIK3CG	PIK3R5
PLCG2	POT1	PRDM1	PTEN	PTK2B	PTPN11	RAD21
RB1	RFC4	RPS15	RUNX1	SETBP1	SF3B1	SMC1A
SMC3	SOCS1	SOCS6	SPI1	SRSF2	STAG2	STAT3
STAT5A	STAT5B	STAT6	SUZ12	*TCF3*	TET2	TNFAIP3
TP53	TP63	U2AF1	UBR5	WHSC1	WHSC1L1	WT1
XPO1	ZEB1	ZRSR2				

Hematologic malignancy fusion analysis of 74 Genes (>5000 selected rearrangements)

ABL1	ABL2	ALK	BCL11B	BCL2	BCL6	BCR
BIRC3	CBFB	CCND1	CCND3	CDK6	CHD1	CHIC2
CIITA	CREBBP	CRLF2	CSF1R	DEK	DUSP22	EBF1
EIF4A1	EPOR	ERG	ETV6	FGFR1	GLIS2	*IKZF1*
IKZF2	IKZF3	JAK2	KAT6A	KLF2	KMT2A	MALT1
MECOM	MKL1	MLF1	MLLT10	MLLT4	MYC	MYH11
NF1	NFKB2	NOTCH1	NTRK3	NUP214	NUP98	P2RY8
PAG1	PAX5	PBX1	PDCD1LG2	PDGFRA	PDGFRB	PICALM
PML	PRDM16	PTK2B	P2PR8	RARA	RBM15	ROS1
RUNX1	RUNX1T1	SEMA6A	SETD2	STIL	TAL1	*TCF3*
TFG	TP63	TYK2	ZCCHC7			

2.8 Case 1: *BCR-ABL1* (Ph) Positive B-ALL

2.8.1 Clinical Presentation and Pathology

A 47-year old female with history of breast cancer 3 years ago was evaluated for the left hip pain and night sweats of one-month duration. She had previously undergone double mastectomy followed by chemotherapy with docetaxel and cyclophosphamide.

Magnetic resonance imaging of left hip showed a 1.6 cm T1 hypointense and T2 hyperintense lesion at left femoral neck. PET/CT scan imaging showed diffuse FDG avidity within axial and proximal appendicular skeleton, focal avid area seen at L femoral neck as well as hypermetabolic mesenteric lymph nodes. She underwent a bone marrow biopsy and CT guided femoral neck biopsy and came to our institution for continued management of her newly diagnosed hematologic malignancy.

At presentation, her laboratory studies showed anemia and thrombocytopenia with white blood cell count (WBC) at 17,600/μL with 29% circulating blasts. The review of bone marrow biopsy revealed B-lymphoblastic leukemia (90% blasts) extensively involving a markedly hypercellular bone marrow. Flow cytometry revealed a classic B-lymphoblastic leukemia immunophenotype, in which the leukemic blasts expressed CD10, CD19, CD20, CD22, CD24, CD34, CD38, HLA-DR, TdT, with no expression of CD117, myeloperoxidase, and other markers tested. Cerebrospinal fluid examination did not show any blasts.

2.8.2 Genomic Evaluation

FISH study revealed the presence of t(9;22)(*BCR/ABL1*) fusion, with minor BCR breakpoint, gain of derivative Ph chromosome, and tetrasomy of chromosome 14. Classical cytogenetic study revealed a complex karyotype as 58,XX, +2, +4,+6, +8, t(9;22)(q34;q11.2), +10, +14, +15, +18, +21, +der(22)t(9;22)(q34;q11.2)[cp5]. The *BCR-ABL1* (p190) fusion transcript was detected at 74.543% by quantitative RT-PCR. No additional genetic testing is warranted in this case given the diagnosis of Ph + ALL (Fig. 2.1) and patient would be treated initially with a combination of tyrosine kinase inhibitor and chemotherapy.

2.9 Case 2: Ph-Like B-ALL

2.9.1 Clinical Presentation and Pathology

The patient was a 44-year-old man who presented with a history of severe abdominal pain lasting for approximately 3 days with a preceding history of tiredness, fatigue, and low energy levels for 3 months. When he was admitted to the hospital for abdominal pain, he was noted to have elevated WBC count of 60,000/

µL with predominantly circulating blasts. His bone marrow biopsy revealed 90% lymphoblasts with expression of CD10, CD20 (subset), CD19, CD22, CD24, CD34, and CD38.

2.9.2 Genomic Evaluation

Cytogenetic study revealed a 46,XY, der(9), t(9;16)(p13;q22), der(16), t(9;16)(p22; q22) karyotype. A FISH study demonstrated loss of *CDKN2A* and translocation of intact *CBFB* to derivative chromosome 9. Sequencing studies were performed using our targeted NGS assay and revealed the following results:

Gene	Genomic Alteration
MLL3	c.13305G > A; p.W4435*
JAK2	c.2600G > A;p.R867Q
P2RY8-CRLF2	Fusion
CRLF2	High expression

2.9.3 Interpretation of NGS Results

The genetic alterations detected by our bioinformatics pipeline were analyzed with multiple disease specific and population databases, review of disease guidelines and published literature, and interpreted as described below:

JAK2: A missense alteration at codon 867 of the JAK2 gene was detected. Mutations of the JAK2 gene, which encodes for a protein tyrosine kinase involved in cytokine receptor signaling, have been found in ~ 10% of B-lymphoblastic leukemia (B-ALL) cases. The p.R867Q alteration detected in this specimen has been previously reported in patients with B-ALL and other solid tumors [51, 105, 106, 143–145].

MLL3: A nonsense alteration at codon 4435 of the MLL3 (also known as KMT2C) gene was detected. Mutations of the MLL3 gene, which encodes a histone lysine methyltransferase and is correlated with tumor suppressor functions, have been found in various hematological malignancies. To our knowledge, the p.W4435* mutation detected in this specimen has never been reported. Furthermore, nonsense mutations like the one in our patient cause premature codon termination and are expected to have a deleterious effect on protein function [100, 146–151].

P2RY8-CRLF2: A fusion of the P2RY8 to CRLF2 gene was detected. Fusions of P2RY8 to CRLF2, are reported to result in deregulated expression of the CRLF2 gene under the control of the P2RY8 promoter and have been found in B-ALL,

Ph-like acute lymphoblastic leukemia (ALL) and Down syndrome associated ALL. Rearrangement of CRLF2 has been associated with mutation of JAK kinases, Latino ethnicity, and poor outcome in pediatric B-ALL. A few studies have reported that increased CRLF2 expression associates with JAK2 mutation as seen in this patient, suggesting that mutant JAK2 and CRLF2 may cooperate in B-ALL pathogenesis. Elevated CRLF2 expression correlates with poor outcome in high-risk B-ALL patients. Adults and children with high-risk CRLF2-rearranged ALL respond poorly to current cytotoxic chemotherapy and suffer unacceptably high rates of relapse; one study reported PI3K/mTOR pathway inhibitors such as rapamycin, PI103, and PP242 also inhibited activated signal transduction and translational machinery proteins of the PI3K/mTOR pathway, suggesting that signal transduction inhibitors targeting this pathway also may have therapeutic relevance for patients with CRLF2-rearranged ALL and merit further preclinical testing. One study reported combined inhibition of JAK/STAT and mTOR pathways by next-generation inhibitors had promising anti-leukemia efficacy in preclinical models of CRFL2-rearranged Ph-like B-ALL [49–58].

These genomic findings of *P2RY8-CRLF2* fusion and *JAK2* mutation helped establish the diagnosis of Ph-like ALL in this case.

The patient underwent induction chemotherapy and attained CR, followed by consolidation on a pediatric type chemotherapy regimen. MRD data during early treatment course was not available. He relapsed 6 months after starting therapy. After treatment with blinatumomab, and subsequently with inotuzumab ozogamicin in combination with chemotherapy, patient entered MRD negative remission and subsequently underwent allogeneic stem cell transplantation using myeloablative radiation-based conditioning. He relapsed 7 months later with extramedullary disease in right submandibular gland without bone marrow involvement and succumbed to his disease [100, 138, 152]. The adverse outcome of Ph-like ALL is illustrated by this case. Whether these cases should undergo allogeneic stem cell transplantation early in disease course remains controversial. It is critical to incorporate the results of MRD analysis in prognostication and decision-making.

2.10 Case 3. T-ALL

2.10.1 Clinical Presentation and Pathology

The patient is a 51-year-old woman who presented with fatigue, malaise, exercise intolerance, and some gastrointestinal complaints. Blood count showed elevated WBC of 224,000/μL, with decreased platelet count of 22,000 μL and hematocrit of 26%. Her clinical history was notable for thyroid cancer for which she underwent surgery followed by radioactive iodine therapy 8 years prior to diagnosis of ALL.

Her diagnostic bone marrow biopsy revealed extensive involvement with T-ALL with 80% blasts. The lymphoblasts expressed CD1a (dim), CD2, cCD3, surface CD3 (dim), CD5, CD7, CD8 (subset), CD24, and CD56 (subset). Blasts were negative for CD4, CD10, CD13, CD16, cCD22, CD33, CD34, HLA-DR, MPO, TCR Alpha–Beta, TCR Gamma-Delta, and TdT. Cytogenetics showed normal female karyotype 46,XX [20]. FISH study demonstrated no assay-specific abnormalities. CSF showed leukemic involvement at diagnosis.

2.10.2 Molecular Genomic Evaluation

Targeted sequencing studies were performed using our NGS-based assay with the following results:

Gene	Genomic Alterations
NOTCH1	**c.7322_7323insTTG; p.D2442***
CCND3	**c.811dup;p.R271Pfs*53**
NUP98-RAP1GDS1	**Fusion**

2.10.3 Interpretation of NGS Mutation Panel Results

The genetic alterations detected by our bioinformatics pipeline were analyzed with multiple disease specific and population databases, review of disease guidelines and published literature and interpreted as described below:

NOTCH1: A nonsense alteration at codon 2442 of the *NOTCH1* gene was detected. As discussed earlier, mutations of the *NOTCH1* gene are among the most common alterations in T-ALL and are found in more than 50% of cases. These mutations affect the heterodimerization domain (HD) or the PEST domain and have been associated with poor outcomes. To our knowledge, the p.D2442* mutation detected in this patient has not been previously reported. However, this alteration is expected to lead to loss of the PEST domain, increased stability of the intracellular domain and activation of the NOTCH1 pathway [91, 153–161].
NUP98-RAP1GDS1: This fusion is one of the known recurrent fusions reported in patients with ALL. *NUP98* fusions are also detected in other human hematopoietic malignancies and associated with poor prognosis [162–172].
CCND3: A frameshift alteration at codon 271 of the *CCND3* gene was detected. The CCND3 gene encodes cyclin D3, which is a critical regulator of cell cycle progression. Mutations of *CCND3* have been found in hematologic malignancies. The p.R271Pfs*53 mutation detected in this specimen has been previously reported in lymphoid disorders. Furthermore, frameshift mutations lead to

premature truncation of the protein and are expected to have a significant deleterious effect [172–175].

This case by definition would be classified as therapy-related ALL given the prior exposure to cytotoxic therapy, i.e., radioactive iodine.

2.10.4 Follow up and Treatment

She was in complete remission with MRD-negative status after induction using a pediatric type chemotherapy regimen. She cleared her CSF with intrathecal chemotherapy. However she was found to have cirrhosis of the liver and hence could not receive the complete course of chemotherapy and ultimately succumbed to liver failure.

References

1. Swerdlow SH, Campo E, Harris NL, Jaffe ES, Pileri SA, Stein H et al (2017) WHO classification of tumors of haematopoietic and lymphoid tissues, revised 4th edn. IARC, Lyon, France
2. Perez-Andreu V, Roberts KG, Xu H et al (2015) A genome-wide association study of susceptibility to acute lymphoblastic leukemia in adolescents and young adults. Blood 125 (4):680–686. https://doi.org/10.1182/blood-2014-09-595744
3. Pullarkat ST, Danley K, Bernstein L, Brynes RK, Cozen W (2009) High lifetime incidence of adult acute lymphoblastic leukemia among Hispanics in California. Cancer Epidemiol Biomarkers Prev 18(2):611–615. https://doi.org/10.1158/1055-9965.EPI-07-2949
4. Hunger SP, Mullighan CG (2015) Acute lymphoblastic leukemia in children. N Engl J Med 373(16):1541–1552. https://doi.org/10.1056/NEJMra1400972
5. Boissel N, Sender LS (2015) Best practices in adolescent and young adult patients with acute lymphoblastic leukemia: a focus on asparaginase. J Adolesc Young Adult Oncol 4(3):118–128. https://doi.org/10.1089/jayao.2015.0014
6. Thomas DA, O'Brien S, Faderl S et al (2010) Chemoimmunotherapy with a modified hyper-CVAD and rituximab regimen improves outcome in de novo Philadelphia chromosome-negative precursor B-lineage acute lymphoblastic leukemia. J Clin Oncol 28 (24):3880–3889. https://doi.org/10.1200/JCO.2009.26.9456
7. Goldstone AH, Richards SM, Lazarus HM et al (2008) In adults with standard-risk acute lymphoblastic leukemia, the greatest benefit is achieved from a matched sibling allogeneic transplantation in first complete remission, and an autologous transplantation is less effective than conventional consolidation/maintenance chemotherapy in all patients: final results of the International ALL Trial (MRC UKALL XII/ECOG E2993). Blood 111(4):1827–1833. https://doi.org/10.1182/blood-2007-10-116582
8. Perez-Andreu V, Roberts KG, Harvey RC et al (2013) Inherited GATA3 variants are associated with Ph-like childhood acute lymphoblastic leukemia and risk of relapse. Nat Genet 45(12):1494–1498. https://doi.org/10.1038/ng.2803
9. Appelbaum FR. Chapter 98: Acute Leukemias in Adults. In: Niederhuber JE, Armitage JO, Dorshow JH, Kastan MB, Tepper JE (eds) (2014) Abeloff's clinical oncology, 5th edn. Elsevier, Philadelphia, PA
10. Jain N, Gurbuxani S, Rhee C, Stock W. Chapter 65: Acute Lymphoblastic Leukemia in Adults. In: Hoffman R, Benz EJ, Silberstein LE, Heslop H, Weitz J, Anastasi J (eds) (2013) Hematology: basic principles and practice, 6th edn. Elsevier, Philadelphia, PA

11. National Cancer Institute (2018) Childhood Acute Lymphoblastic Leukemia Treatment (PDQ®). www.cancer.gov/types/leukemia/patient/child-all-treatment-pdq. Accessed 19 July 2018
12. National Cancer Institute (2018) SEER Cancer Stat Facts: Acute Lymphocytic Leukemia (ALL). https://seer.cancer.gov/statfacts/html/alyl.html. Accessed July 18 2018
13. Ribera JM (2018) Therapy-related acute lymphoblastic leukemia. Haematologica 103 (10):1581–1583. https://doi.org/10.3324/haematol.2018.200311
14. Moorman AV (2012) The clinical relevance of chromosomal and genomic abnormalities in B-cell precursor acute lymphoblastic leukaemia. Blood Rev 26(3)
15. Moorman AV, Chilton L, Wilkinson J, Ensor HM, Bown N, Proctor SJ (2010) A population-based cytogenetic study of adults with acute lymphoblastic leukaemia. Blood 115 (2):206–214
16. Gleißner B, Gökbuget N, Bartram CR, Janssen B, Rieder H, Janssen JWG, Fonatsch C, Heyll A, Voliotis D, Beck J, Lipp T, Munzert G, Maurer J, Hoelzer D, Thiel E, the German Multicenter Trials of Adult Acute Lymphoblastic Leukemia Study Group (2002) Leading prognostic relevance of the BCR-ABL translocation in adult acute B-lineage lymphoblastic leukemia: a prospective study of the German Multicenter Trial Group and confirmed polymerase chain reaction analysis. Blood 99(5):1536–1543
17. Cytogenetic abnormalities in adult acute lymphoblastic leukemia: correlations with hematologic findings outcome (1996) A Collaborative Study of the Group Français de Cytogénétique Hématologique [published correction appears in Blood 1996 Oct 1;88 (7):2818]. Blood 87(8):3135–3142
18. Westbrook CA, Hooberman AL, Spino C et al (1992) Clinical significance of the BCR-ABL fusion gene in adult acute lymphoblastic leukemia: a cancer and leukemia group B Study (8762). Blood 80(12):2983–2990
19. Sattler M, Griffin JD (2001) Mechanisms of transformation by the BCR/ABL oncogene. Int J Hematol 73(3):278–291
20. Harrison CJ, Moorman AV, Barber KE et al (2005) Interphase molecular cytogenetic screening for chromosomal abnormalities of prognostic significance in childhood acute lymphoblastic leukaemia: a UK cancer cytogenetics group study. Br J Haematol 129(4):520–530. https://doi.org/10.1111/j.1365-2141.2005.05497
21. Woo HY, Kim DW, Park H, Seong KW, Koo HH, Kim SH (2005) Molecular cytogenetic analysis of gene rearrangements in childhood acute lymphoblastic leukemia. J Korean Med Sci 20(1):36–41. https://doi.org/10.3346/jkms.2005.20.1.36
22. Cimino G, Elia L, Rapanotti MC et al (2000) A prospective study of residual-disease monitoring of the ALL1/AF4 transcript in patients with t(4;11) acute lymphoblastic leukemia. Blood 95(1):96–101
23. Golub TR, Barker GF, Bohlander SK et al (1995) Fusion of the TEL gene on 12p13 to the AML1 gene on 21q22 in acute lymphoblastic leukemia. Proc Natl Acad Sci U S A 92 (11):4917–4921. https://doi.org/10.1073/pnas.92.11.4917
24. Borkhardt A, Cazzaniga G, Viehmann S et al (1997) Incidence and clinical relevance of TEL/AML1 fusion genes in childrenwith acute lymphoblastic leukemia enrolled in the German and Italian multicenter therapy trials. Associazione Italiana Ematologia Oncologia Pediatrica and the Berlin-Frankfurt-Münster Study Group. Blood 90(2):571–577
25. Rambaldi A, Attuati V, Bassan R et al (1996) Molecular diagnosis and clinical relevance of t (9;22), t(4;11) and t(1; 19) chromosome abnormalities in a consecutive group of 141 adult patients with acute lymphoblastic leukemia. Leuk Lymphoma 21(5–6):457–466
26. Devaraj PE, Foroni L, Janossy G, Hoffbrand AV, Secker-Walker LM (1995) Expression of the E2A-PBX1 fusion transcripts in t(1;19)(q23;p13) and der(19)t(1;19) at diagnosis and in remission of acute lymphoblastic leukemia with different B lineage immunophenotypes. Leukemia 9(5):821–825

27. V, Zenger M, Schnittger S et al (2014) Acute lymphoblastic leukemia with low hypodiploid/near triploid karyotype is a specific clinical entity and exhibits a very high TP53 mutation frequency of 93%. Genes Chromosomes Cancer 53(6):524–536

28. Ross ME, Zhou X, Song G et al (2003) Classification of pediatric acute lymphoblastic leukemia by gene expression profiling. Blood 102(8):2951–2959

29. Den Boer ML, van Slegtenhorst M, De Menezes RX et al (2009) A subtype of childhood acute lymphoblastic leukaemia with poor treatment outcome: a genome-wide classification study. Lancet Oncol 10(2):125–134. https://doi.org/10.1016/S1470-2045(08)70339-5

30. Comeaux EQ, Mullighan CG (2017) TP53 mutations in hypodiploid acute lymphoblastic leukemia. Cold Spring Harb Perspect Med 7(3):a026286

31. Holmfeldt L, Wei L, Diaz-Flores E et al (2013) The genomic landscape of hypodiploid acute lymphoblastic leukemia. Nat Genet 45(3):242–252

32. Grimaldi JC, Meeker TC (1989) The t(5;14) chromosomal translocation in a case of acute lymphocytic leukemia joins the interleukin-3 gene to the immunoglobulin heavy chain gene. Blood 73(8):2081–2085

33. Harrison CJ, Moorman AV, Schwab C et al (2014) An international study of intrachromosomal amplification of chromosome 21 (iAMP21): cytogenetic characterization and outcome. Leukemia 28(5):1015–1021

34. Heerema NA, Carroll AJ, Devidas M et al (2013) Intrachromosomal amplification of chromosome 21 is associated with inferior outcomes in children with acute lymphoblastic leukemia treated in contemporary standard-risk children's oncology group studies: a report from the children's oncology group. J Clin Oncol 31(27):3397–3402

35. Afkhami M (2019) Philadelphia-like lymphoblastic leukemia: approach to testing in clinical laboratories for diagnosis, prognosis, and therapeutic risk assessment. Adv Mol Pathol 2 (1):59–64

36. Kang H, Chen IM, Wilson CS et al (2010) Gene expression classifiers for relapse-free survival and minimal residual disease improve risk classification and outcome prediction in pediatric B-precursor acute lymphoblastic leukemia. Blood 115(7):1394–1405

37. Mullighan CG, Goorha S, Radtke I et al (2007) Genome-wide analysis of genetic alterations in acute lymphoblastic leukaemia. Nature 446:758–764

38. Roberts KG, Gu Z, Payne-Turner D et al (2017) High frequency and poor outcome of Philadelphia chromosome-like acute lymphoblastic leukemia in adults. J Clin Oncol 35:394–401

39. Tasian SK, Hurtz C, Wertheim GB et al (2017) High incidence of Philadelphia chromosome-like acute lymphoblastic leukemia in older adults with B-ALL. Leukemia 31:981–984

40. Roberts KG, Li Y, Payne-turner D et al (2014) Targetable kinase activating lesions in Ph-like acute lymphoblastic leukemia. N Engl J Med 371(11):1005–1015

41. Reshmi SC, Harvey RC, Roberts KG et al (2017) Targetable kinase gene fusions in high-risk B-ALL: a study from the children's oncology group. Blood 129(25):3352–3361

42. Walsh KM, De smith AJ, Chokkalingam AP et al (2013) GATA3 risk alleles are associated with ancestral components in Hispanic children with ALL. Blood 122(19):3385–3387

43. Jain N, Roberts KG, Jabbour E et al (2017) Ph-like acute lymphoblastic leukemia: a high-risk subtype in adults. Blood 129:572–581

44. Wells J, Jain N, Konopleva M (2017) Philadelphia chromosome like acute lymphoblastic leukemia: progress in a new cancer subtype. Clin AdvHematol Oncol 15(7):554–561

45. Tasian SK, Doral MY, Borowitz MJ et al (2012) Aberrant STAT5 and PI3K/mTOR pathway signaling occurs in human CRLF2-rearranged B-precursor acute lymphoblastic leukemia. Blood 120(4):833–842

46. Russell LJ, Capasso M, Vater I et al (2009) Deregulated expression of cytokine receptor gene, CRLF2, is involved in lymphoid transformation in B-cell precursor acute lymphoblastic leukemia. Blood 114(13):2688–2698

47. Palmi C, Vendramini E, Silvestri D et al (2012) Poor prognosis for P2RY8-CRLF2 fusion but not for CRLF2 over-expression in children with intermediate risk B-cell precursor acute lymphoblastic leukemia. Leukemia 26(10):2245–2253
48. Cario G, Zimmermann M, Romey R et al (2010) Presence of the P2RY8-CRLF2 rearrangement is associated with a poor prognosis in non-high-risk precursor B-cell acute lymphoblastic leukemia in children treated according to the ALL-BFM 2000 protocol. Blood 115(26):5393–5397
49. Harvey RC, Mullighan CG, Chen IM et al (2010) Rearrangement of CRLF2 is associated with mutation of JAK kinases, alteration of IKZF1, Hispanic/Latino ethnicity, and a poor outcome in pediatric B-progenitor acute lymphoblastic leukemia. Blood 115(26):5312–5321
50. Yamashita Y, Shimada A, Yamada T et al (2013) IKZF1 and CRLF2 gene alterations correlate with poor prognosis in Japanese BCR-ABL1-negative high-risk B-cell precursor acute lymphoblastic leukemia. Pediatr Blood Cancer 60(10):1587–1592
51. Roll JD, Reuther GW (2010) CRLF2 and JAK2 in B-progenitor acute lymphoblastic leukemia: a novel association in oncogenesis. Cancer Res 70(19):7347–7352
52. Yoda A, Yoda Y, Chiaretti S et al (2010) Functional screening identifies CRLF2 in precursor B-cell acute lymphoblastic leukemia. Proc Natl Acad Sci USA 107(1):252–257
53. Van bodegom D, Zhong J, Kopp N et al (2012) Differences in signaling through the B-cell leukemia oncoprotein CRLF2 in response to TSLP and through mutant JAK2. Blood 120 (14):2853–2863
54. Sarno J, Savino AM, Buracchi C et al (2018) SRC/ABL inhibition disrupts CRLF2-driven signaling to induce cell death in B-cell acute lymphoblastic leukemia. Oncotarget 9 (33):22872–22885
55. Tasian SK, Teachey DT, Li Y et al (2017) Potent efficacy of combined PI3K/mTOR and JAK or ABL inhibition in murine xenograft models of Ph-like acute lymphoblastic leukemia. Blood 129(2):177–187
56. Maude SL, Tasian SK, Vincent T et al (2012) Targeting JAK1/2 and mTOR in murine xenograft models of Ph-like acute lymphoblastic leukemia. Blood 120(17):3510–3518
57. Zhang Q, Shi C, Han L et al (2018) Inhibition of mTORC1/C2 signaling improves anti-leukemia efficacy of JAK/STAT blockade in rearranged and/or driven Philadelphia chromosome-like acute B-cell lymphoblastic leukemia. Oncotarget 9(8):8027–8041
58. Mullighan CG (2011) New strategies in acute lymphoblastic leukemia: translating advances in genomics into clinical practice. Clin Cancer Res 17(3):396–400
59. Boer JM, Den boer ML (2017) BCR-ABL1-like acute lymphoblastic leukaemia: from bench to bedside. Eur J Cancer 82:203–218
60. Iacobucci I, Li Y, Roberts KG et al (2016) Truncating erythropoietin receptor rearrangements in acute lymphoblastic leukemia. Cancer Cell 29(2):186–200
61. Molteni CG, Te kronnie G, Bicciato S et al (2010) PTPN11 mutations in childhood acute lymphoblastic leukemia occur as a secondary event associated with high hyperdiploidy. Leukemia 24(1).232–235
62. Yamamoto T, Isomura M, Xu Y et al (2006) PTPN11, RAS and FLT3 mutations in childhood acute lymphoblastic leukemia. Leuk Res 30(9):1085–1089
63. Tartaglia M, Martinelli S, Cazzaniga G et al (2004) Genetic evidence for lineage-related and differentiation stage-related contribution of somatic PTPN11 mutations to leukemogenesis in childhood acute leukemia. Blood 104(2):307–313
64. Dahéron L, Brizard F, Millot F, Cividin M, Lacotte L, Guilhot F, Brizard A (2002) E2A/HLF fusion gene in an acute lymphoblastic leukemia patient with disseminated intravascular coagulation and a normal karyotype. Hematol J 3(3):153–156. https://doi.org/10.1038/sj.thj.6200169 PMID: 12111652
65. Medeiros BC (2009) Deletion of IKZF1 and prognosis in acute lymphoblastic leukemia. N Engl J Med 360(17):1787
66. Marke R, Van leeuwen FN, Scheijen B (2018) The many faces of IKZF1 in B-cell precursor acute lymphoblastic leukemia. Haematologica 103(4):565–574

67. Yao QM, Liu KY, Gale RP et al (2016) Prognostic impact of IKZF1 deletion in adults with common B-cell acute lymphoblastic leukemia. BMC Cancer 16:269

68. Lana T, De lorenzo P, Bresolin S et al (2015) Refinement of IKZF1 status in pediatric Philadelphia-positive acute lymphoblastic leukemia. Leukemia 29(10):2107–2110

69. Mullighan CG (2012) The molecular genetic makeup of acute lymphoblastic leukemia. Hematol Am Soc Hematol Educ Program 389–396

70. Mullighan CG, Su X, Zhang J et al (2009) Deletion of IKZF1 and prognosis in acute lymphoblastic leukemia. N Engl J Med 360(5):470–480

71. Kastner P, Dupuis A, Gaub MP, Herbrecht R, Lutz P, Chan S (2013) Function of Ikaros as a tumor suppressor in B cell acute lymphoblastic leukemia. Am J Blood Res 3(1):1–13

72. Iacobucci I, Lonetti A, Messa F et al (2008) Expression of spliced oncogenic Ikaros isoforms in Philadelphia-positive acute lymphoblastic leukemia patients treated with tyrosine kinase inhibitors: implications for a new mechanism of resistance. Blood 112(9):3847–3855

73. Iacobucci I, Iraci N, Messina M et al (2012) IKAROS deletions dictate a unique gene expression signature in patients with adult B-cell acute lymphoblastic leukemia. PLoS ONE 7(7):e40934

74. Sun L, Goodman PA, Wood CM et al (1999) Expression of aberrantly spliced oncogenic ikaros isoforms in childhood acute lymphoblastic leukemia. J Clin Oncol 17(12):3753–3766

75. Beldjord K, Chevret S, Asnafi V et al (2014) Oncogenetics and minimal residual disease are independent outcome predictors in adult patients with acute lymphoblastic leukemia. Blood 123(24):3739–3749

76. Goldberg JM, Silverman LB, Levy DE et al (2003) Childhood T-cell acute lymphoblastic leukemia: the Dana-Farber Cancer Institute acute lymphoblastic leukemia consortium experience. J Clin Oncol 21(19):3616–3622

77. Willemse MJ, Seriu T, Hettinger K et al (2002) Detection of minimal residual disease identifies differences in treatment response between T-ALL and precursor B-ALL. Blood 99 (12):4386–4393

78. Schrappe M, Valsecchi MG, Bartram CR et al (2011) Late MRD response determines relapse risk overall and in subsets of childhood T-cell ALL: results of the AIEOP-BFM-ALL 2000 study. Blood 118(8):2077–2084

79. Morel P, Lepage E, Brice P et al (1992) Prognosis and treatment of lymphoblastic lymphoma in adults: a report on 80 patients. J Clin Oncol 10(7):1078–1085

80. Patrick K, Wade R, Goulden N et al (2014) Outcome for children and young people with early T-cell precursor acute lymphoblastic leukaemia treated on a contemporary protocol, UKALL 2003. Br J Haematol 166:421–424 PMID:24708207

81. Wood BL, Winter SS, Dunsmore KP et al (2014) T-lymphoblastic leukemia (T-ALL) shows excellent outcome, lack of significance of the early thymic precursor (ETP) immune-phenotype, and validation of the prognostic value of end-induction minimal residual disease (MRD) in children's oncology group (COG) study AALL0434. Blood 124(21):1

82. Guo RJ, Bahmanyar M, Minden MD et al (2016) CD33, not early precursor T-cell phenotype, is associated with adverse outcome in adult T-cell acute lymphoblastic leukemia. Br J Haematol 172:823–825 PMID:26123477

83. Robertson PB, Neiman RS, Worapong-paiboon S et al (1997) 013 (CD99) positivity in hematologic proliferations correlates with TdT positivity. Mod Pathol 10:277–282 PMID:9110287

84. Chetty R, Pulford K, Jones M et al (1995) SCL/TAL-1 expression in T-acute lymphoblastic leukemia: an immunohistochemical and genotypic study. Hum Pathol 26:994–998 PMID:7672800

85. Delabesse E, Bernard M, Meyer V et al (1998) TAL1 expression does not occur in the majority of T-ALL blasts. Br J Haematol 102:449–457 PMID:9695959

86. Pilozzi E, Pulford K, Jones M et al (1998) Co-expression of CD79a (JCB117) and CD3 by lymphoblastic lymphoma. J Pathol186:140–143. PMID:9924428

87. Khalidi HS, Chang KL, Medeiros LJ et al (1999) Acute lymphoblastic leukemia. Survey of immunophenotype, French-American-British classification, frequency of myeloid antigen expression, and karyotypic abnormaiities in 210 pediatric and adult cases. Am J Ciin Pathol 111:467–476. PMiD:10191766

88. Uckun FM, Bather HN, Gaynon PS et al (1997) Clinical features and treatment outcome of children with myeloid antigen positive acute lymphoblastic leukemia: a report from the children's cancer group. Blood 90:28–35. PMID:9207434

89. Paietta E, Ferrando AA, Neuberg D et al (2004) Activating FLT3 mutations in CD117/KIT (+) T-cell acute lymphoblastic leukemias. Blood 104:558–560. PMID:15044257

90. Bene MC, Castoldi G, Knapp W et al (1995) Proposals for the immunological classification of acute leukemias. Leukemia 9:1783–1786, PMID:7564526

91. Weng AP, Ferrando AA, Lee W et al (2004) Activating mutations of NOTCH1 in human T cell acute lymphoblastic leukemia. Science 306:269–271. PMID:15472075

92. Weng AP, Millholland JM, Yashiro-Ohtani Y et al (2006) c-Myc is an important direct target of Notch1 in T-cell acute lymphoblastic leukemia/lymphoma. Genes Dev 20:2096–2109. PMID:16847353

93. Zhu YM, Zhao WL, Fu JF et al (2006) NOTCH1 mutations in T-cell acute lymphoblastic leukemia: prognostic significance and implication in multifactorial leukemogenesis. Clin Cancer Res 12:3043–3049, PMID:16707600

94. Malyukova A, Dohda T, von der Lehr N et al (2007) The tumor suppressor gene hCDC4 is frequently mutated in human T-cell acute lymphoblastic leukemia with functional consequences for Notch signaling. Cancer Res 67:5611–5616. PMID:17575125

95. Van vlierberghe P, Palomero T, Khiabanian H et al (2010) PHF6 mutations in T-cell acute lymphoblastic leukemia. Nat Genet 42(4):338–342

96. Yoo NJ, Kim YR, Lee SH (2012) Somatic mutation of PHF6 gene in T-cell acute lymphoblatic leukemia, acute myelogenous leukemia and hepatocellular carcinoma. Acta Oncol 51(1):107–111

97. Wang Q, Qiu H, Jiang H et al (2011) Mutations of PHF6 are associated with mutations of NOTCH1, JAK1 and rearrangement of SET-NUP214 in T-cell acute lymphoblastic leukemia. Haematologica 96(12):1808–1814

98. Li M, Xiao L, Xu J et al (2016) Co-existence of PHF6 and NOTCH1 mutations in adult T-cell acute lymphoblastic leukemia. Oncol Lett 12(1):16–22

99. Van vlierberghe P, Ferrando A (2012) The molecular basis of T cell acute lymphoblastic leukemia. J Clin Invest 122(10):3398–3406

100. Spinella JF, Cassart P, Richer C et al (2016) Genomic characterization of pediatric T-cell acute lymphoblastic leukemia reveals novel recurrent driver mutations. Oncotarget 7 (40):65485–65503

101. Zhou X, Gu Y, Han Q, Soliman M, Song C, Ge Z (2017) Coexistence of EZH2, NOTCH1, IL7R, and PHF6 mutations in Adult T-cell acute lymphoblastic leukemia. Turk J Haematol 34(4).366–368

102. Mori T, Nagata Y, Makishima H et al (2016) Somatic PHF6 mutations in 1760 cases with various myeloid neoplasms. Leukemia 122(21):2514

103. Van Vlierberghe P, Patel J, Abdel-Wahab O et al (2011) PHF6 mutations in adult acute myeloid leukemia. Leukemia 25(1):130–134

104. Flex E, Petrangeli V, Stella L et al (2008) Somatically acquired JAK1 mutations in adult acute lymphoblastic leukemia. J Exp Med 205(4):751–758

105. Mullighan CG, Zhang J, Harvey RC et al (2009) JAK mutations in high-risk childhood acute lymphoblastic leukemia. Proc Natl Acad Sci USA 106(23):9414–9418

106. Mullighan CG (2008) JAK2- a new player in acute lymphoblastic leukemia. Lancet 372 (9648):1448–1450

107. Greenplate A, Wang K, Tripathi RM et al (2018) Genomic profiling of T-cell neoplasms reveals frequent JAK1 and JAK3 mutations with clonal evasion from targeted therapies. JCO Precis Oncol

108. Hornakova T, Chiaretti S, Lemaire MM et al (2010) ALL-associated JAK1 mutations confer hypersensitivity to the antiproliferative effect of type I interferon. Blood 115(16):3287–3295
109. Coustan-Smith E, Mullighan CG, Onciu M et al (2009) Early T-cell precursor leukaemia: a subtype of very high-risk acute lymphoblastic leukaemia. Lancet Oncol 10:147–156. PMID:19147408
110. Zhang J, Ding L, Hoimfeldt L et al (2012) The genetic basis of early T-cell precursor acute lymphoblastic leukaemia. Nature 481:157–163. PMID:22237106
111. Van Vlierberghe P, Ambesi-Impiombato A, Perez-Garcia A et al (2011) ETV6 mutations in early immature human T cell leukemias. J Exp Med 208:2571–2579. PMID:22162831
112. Neumann M, Coskun E, Fransecky L et al (2013) FLT3 mutations in early T-cell precursor ALL characterize a stem cell like leukemia and imply the clinical use of tyrosine kinase inhibitors. PLoS One 8:e53190. PMID:23359050
113. Neumann M, Heesch S, Schlee C et al (2013) Whole-exome sequencing in adult ETP- ALL reveals a high rate of DNMT3A mutations. Blood 121:4749–4752. PMID:23603912
114. Graux C, Cools J, Michaux L et al (2006) Cytogenetics and molecular genetics of T-cell acute lymphoblastic leukemia: from thymocyte to lymphoblast. Leukemia 20:1496–1510. PMID:16826225
115. Han X, Bueso-Ramos CE (2007) Precursor T-cell acute lymphoblastic leukemia/lymphoblastic lymphoma and acute biphenotypic leukemias. Am J Clin Pathol 127:528–544. PMID:17369128
116. Pilozzi E, Muller-Hermelink HK, Falini B et al (1999) Gene rearrangements in T-cell lymphoblastic lymphoma. J Pathol 188:267–270. PMID:10419594
117. Szczepaiiski T, Pongers-Willemse MJ, Langerak AW et al (1999) Ig heavy chain gene rearrangements in T-cell acute lymphoblastic leukemia exhibit predominant DH6-19 and DH7-27 gene usage, can result in complete V-D-J rearrangements, and are rare in T-cell receptor alpha beta lineage. Blood 93:4079–4085. PMID:10361104
118. De Keersmaecker K, Marynen P, Cools J (2005) Genetic insights in the pathogenesis of T-cell acute lymphoblastic leukemia. Haematologica 90:1116–1127. PMID:16079112
119. Meijerink JP (2010) Genetic rearrangements in relation to immunophenotype and outcome in T-cell acute lymphoblastic leukaemia. Best Pract Res Clin Haematol 23:307–318. PMID:21112032
120. Van Vlierberghe P, Pieters R, Beverloo HB et al (2008) Molecular-genetic insights in paediatric T-cell acute lymphoblastic leukaemia. Br J Haematol 143:153–168. PMID:18691165
121. Ferrando AA, Neuberg DS, Staunton J et al (2002) Gene expression signatures define novel oncogenic pathways in T cell acute lymphoblastic leukemia. Cancer Cell 1:75–87. PMID:12086890
122. Kumon K, Kobayashi H, Maseki N et al (1999) Mixed-lineage leukemia with t(10;11)(p13; q21): an analysis of AF10-CALM and CALM-AF10 fusion mRNAs and clinical features. Genes Chromosomes Cancer 25(1):33–39
123. Carlson KM, Vignon C, Bohlander S, Martinez-climent JA, Le beau MM, Rowley JD (2000) Identification and molecular characterization of CALM/AF10fusion products in T cell acute lymphoblastic leukemia and acute myeloid leukemia. Leukemia 14(1):100–104
124. Ben abdelali R, Asnafi V, Petit A et al (2013) The prognosis of CALM-AF10-positive adult T-cell acute lymphoblastic leukemias depends on the stage of maturation arrest. Haematologica 98(11):1711–1717
125. Borel C, Dastugue N, Cances-lauwers V et al (2012) PICALM-MLLT10 acute myeloid leukemia: a French cohort of 18 patients. Leuk Res 36(11):1365–1369
126. Lo nigro L, Mirabile E, Tumino M et al (2013) Detection of PICALM-MLLT10 (CALM-AF10) and outcome in children with T-lineage acute lymphoblastic leukemia. Leukemia 27(12):2419–2421

127. Narita M, Shimizu K, Hayashi Y et al (1999) Consistent detection of CALM-AF10 chimaeric transcripts in haematological malignancies with t(10;11)(p13;q14) and identification of novel transcripts. Br J Haematol 105(4):928–937
128. Dreyling MH, Martinez-climent JA, Zheng M, Mao J, Rowley JD, Bohlander SK (1996) The t(10;11)(p13;q14) in the U937 cell line results in the fusion of the AF10 gene and CALM, encoding a new member of the AP-3 clathrin assembly protein family. Proc Natl Acad Sci USA 93(10):4804–4809
129. Roberts KG, Li Y, Payne-turner D et al (2014) Targetable kinase-activating lesions in Ph-like acute lymphoblastic leukemia. N Engl J Med 371(11):1005–1015
130. Graux C, Cools J, Melotte C et al (2004) Fusion of NUP214 to ABL1 on amplified episomes in T-cell acute lymphoblastic leukemia. Nat Genet 36(10):1084–1089
131. Duployez N, Grzych G, Ducourneau B et al (2016) NUP214-ABL1 fusion defines a rare subtype of B-cell precursor acute lymphoblastic leukemia that could benefit from tyrosine kinase inhibitors. Haematologica 101(4):e133–e134
132. Giacomini CP, Sun S, Varma S et al (2013) Breakpoint analysis of transcriptional and genomic profiles uncovers novel gene fusions spanning multiple human cancer types. PLoS Genet 9(4):e1003464
133. Burmeister T, Gökbuget N, Reinhardt R, Rieder H, Hoelzer D, Schwartz S (2006) NUP214-ABL1 in adult T-ALL: the GMALL study group experience. Blood 108(10):3556–3559
134. De keersmaecker K, Porcu M, Cox L et al (2014) NUP214-ABL1-mediated cell proliferation in T-cell acute lymphoblastic leukemia is dependent on the LCK kinase and various interacting proteins. Haematologica 99(1):85–93
135. Akin C, Fumo G, Yavuz AS et al (2004) A novel form of mastocytosis associated with a transmembrane c-kit mutation and response to imatinib. Blood 103:3222–3225. PMID:15070706
136. Roberts KG, Reshmi SC, Harvey RC et al (2018) Genomic and outcome analyses of Ph-like ALL in NCI standard-risk patients: a report from the children's oncology group. Blood 132:815–824
137. Chiaretti S, Messina M, Foà R (2019) BCR/ABL1-like acute lymphoblastic leukemia: how to diagnose and treat? Cancer 125(2):194–204
138. Stein AS, Palmer JM, O'Donnell MR et al (2009) Reduced-intensity conditioning followed by peripheral blood stem cell transplantation for adult patients with high-risk acute lymphoblastic leukemia. Biol Blood Marrow Transplant 15(11):1407–1414
139. Chalandon Y, Thomas X, Hayette S et al (2015) Randomized study of reduced-intensity chemotherapy combined with imatinib in adults with Ph-positive acute lymphoblastic leukemia [published correction appears in Blood. 2015 Sep 3;126(10):1261]. Blood 125 (24):3711–3719
140. Mohty M, Labopin M, Volin L et al (2010) Reduced-intensity versus conventional myeloablative conditioning allogeneic stem cell transplantation for patients with acute lymphoblastic leukemia: a retrospective study from the European Group for blood and marrow transplantation. Blood 116(22):4439–4443
141. Kantarjian H, Thomas D, Jorgensen J et al (2013) Results of inotuzumab ozogamicin, a CD22 monoclonal antibody, in refractory and relapsed acute lymphocytic leukemia. Cancer 119(15):2728–2736
142. Thomas DA, Faderl S, O'Brien S et al (2006) Chemoimmunotherapy with hyper-CVAD plus rituximab for the treatment of adult Burkitt and Burkitt-type lymphoma or acute lymphoblastic leukemia. Cancer 106(7):1569–1580
143. Steeghs EMP, Jerchel IS, De goffau-nobel W et al (2017) JAK2 aberrations in childhood B-cell precursor acute lymphoblastic leukemia. Oncotarget 8(52):89923–89938
144. Roncero AM, López-nieva P, Cobos-fernández MA et al (2016) Contribution of JAK2 mutations to T-cell lymphoblastic lymphoma development. Leukemia 30(1):94–103

145. Sadras T, Heatley SL, Kok CH et al (2017) A novel somatic JAK2 kinase-domain mutation in pediatric acute lymphoblastic leukemia with rapid on-treatment development of LOH. Cancer Genet 216–217:86–90

146. Hu D, Shilatifard A (2016) Epigenetics of hematopoiesis and hematological malignancies. Genes Dev 30(18):2021–2041

147. Ruault M, Brun ME, Ventura M, Roizès G, De sario A (2002) MLL3, a new human member of the TRX/MLL gene family, maps to 7q36, a chromosome region frequently deleted in myeloid leukaemia. Gene 284(1–2):73–81

148. Rao RC, Dou Y (2015) Hijacked in cancer: the KMT2 (MLL) family of methyltransferases. Nat Rev Cancer 15(6):334–346

149. Chen C, Liu Y, Rappaport AR et al (2014) MLL3 is a haploinsufficient 7q tumor suppressor in acute myeloid leukemia. Cancer Cell 25(5):652–665

150. Ford DJ, Dingwall AK (2015) The cancer COMPASS: navigating the functions of MLL complexes in cancer. Cancer Genet 208(5):178–191

151. Kayser S, Feszler M, Krzykalla J et al (2017) Clinical impact of KMT2C and SPRY4 expression levels in intensively treated younger adult acute myeloid leukemia patients. Eur J Haematol 99(6):544–552

152. Malecki MJ, Sanchez-Irizarry C, Mitchell JL et al (2006) Leukemia-associated mutations within the NOTCH1 heterodimerization domain fall into at least two distinct mechanistic classes. Mol Cell Biol 26(12):4642–4651

153. Huh HJ, Lee SH, Yoo KH et al (2013) Gene mutation profiles and prognostic implications in Korean patients with T-lymphoblastic leukemia. Ann Hematol 92(5):635–644

154. Neumann M, Vosberg S, Schlee C et al (2015) Mutational spectrum of adult T-ALL. Oncotarget 6(5):2754–2766

155. Weng AP, Ferrando AA, Lee W et al (2004) Activating mutations of NOTCH1 in human T cell acute lymphoblastic leukemia. Science 306(5694):269–271

156. Villamor N, Conde L, Martínez-trillos A et al (2013) NOTCH1 mutations identify a genetic subgroup of chronic lymphocytic leukemia patients with high risk of transformation and poor outcome. Leukemia 27(5):1100–1106

157. Gianfelici V (2012) Activation of the NOTCH1 pathway in chronic lymphocytic leukemia. Haematologica 97(3):328–330

158. Weissmann S, Roller A, Jeromin S et al (2013) Prognostic impact and landscape of NOTCH1 mutations in chronic lymphocytic leukemia (CLL): a study on 852 patients. Leukemia 27(12):2393–2396

159. Willander K, Dutta RK, Ungerbäck J et al (2013) NOTCH1 mutations influence survival in chronic lymphocytic leukemia patients. BMC Cancer 13:274

160. Nakamura T, Largaespada DA, Lee MP et al (1996) Fusion of the nucleoporin gene NUP98 to HOXA9 by the chromosome translocation t(7;11)(p15;p15) in human myeloid leukaemia. Nat Genet 12(2):154–158

161. Slape C, Aplan PD (2004) The role of NUP98 gene fusions in hematologic malignancy. Leuk Lymphoma 45(7):1341–1350

162. Kobzev YN, Martinez-climent J, Lee S, Chen J, Rowley JD (2004) Analysis of translocations that involve the NUP98 gene in patients with 11p15 chromosomal rearrangements. Genes Chromosomes Cancer 41(4):339–352

163. Gough SM, Slape CI, Aplan PD (2011) NUP98 gene fusions and hematopoietic malignancies: common themes and new biologic insights. Blood 118(24):6247–6257

164. Nakamura T, Yamazaki Y, Hatano Y, Miura I (1999) NUP98 is fused to PMX1 homeobox gene in human acute myelogenous leukemia with chromosome translocation t(1;11)(q23;p15). Blood 94(2):741–747

165. Petit A, Radford I, Waill MC, Romana S, Berger R (2008) NUP98-NSD1 fusion by insertion in acute myeloblastic leukemia. Cancer Genet Cytogenet 180(1):43–46

166. Hollink IH, Van den heuvel-eibrink MM, Arentsen-peters ST et al (2011) NUP98/NSD1 characterizes a novel poor prognostic group in acute myeloid leukemia with a distinct HOX gene expression pattern. Blood 118(13):3645–3656
167. Hussey DJ, Nicola M, Moore S, Peters GB, Dobrovic A (1999) The (4;11)(q21;p15) translocation fuses the NUP98 and RAP1GDS1 genes and is recurrent in T-cell acute lymphocytic leukemia. Blood 94(6):2072–2079
168. Mecucci C, La starza R, Negrini M et al (2000) t(4;11)(q21;p15) translocation involving NUP98 and RAP1GDS1 genes: characterization of a new subset of T acute lymphoblastic leukaemia. Br J Haematol 109(4):788–793
169. Cimino G, Sprovieri T, Rapanotti MC, Foà R, Mecucci C, Mandelli F (2001) Molecular evaluation of the NUP98/RAP1GDS1 gene frequency in adults with T-acute lymphoblastic leukemia. Haematologica 86(4):436–437
170. Van zutven LJ, Onen E, Velthuizen SC et al (2006) Identification of NUP98 abnormalities in acute leukemia: JARID1A (12p13) as a new partner gene. Genes Chromosomes Cancer 45 (5):437–446
171. Sonoki T, Harder L, Horsman DE et al (2001) Cyclin D3 is a target gene of t(6;14)(p21.1; q32.3) of mature B-cell malignancies. Blood 98(9):2837–2844
172. Filipits M, Jaeger U, Pohl G et al (2002) Cyclin D3 is a predictive and prognostic factor in diffuse large B-cell lymphoma. Clin Cancer Res 8(3):729–733
173. Curiel-olmo S, Mondéjar R, Almaraz C et al (2017) Splenic diffuse red pulp small B-cell lymphoma displays increased expression of cyclin D3 and recurrent CCND3 mutations. Blood 129(8):1042–1045
174. Rohde M, Bonn BR, Zimmermann M et al (2017) Relevance of ID3-TCF3-CCND3 pathway mutations in pediatric aggressive B-cell lymphoma treated according to the non-Hodgkin Lymphoma Berlin-Frankfurt-Münster protocols. Haematologica 102(6):1091–1098
175. Morin RD, Assouline S, Alcaide M et al (2016) Genetic landscapes of relapsed and refractory diffuse large B-cell lymphomas. Clin Cancer Res 22(9):2290–2300

Acute Promyelocytic Leukemia: Update on Risk Stratification and Treatment Practices

3

Amandeep Salhotra and Matthew Mei

3.1 Background and Epidemiology

Acute promyelocytic leukemia (APL) is a rare but highly curable form of acute myeloid leukemia (AML) whose genetic hallmark is the balanced reciprocal translocation t(15;17)(q22;q12) which fuses the promyelocytic leukemia (*PML*) and retinoic acid receptor alpha (*RARα*) genes [1, 2]. It is a rare disease and accounts for 5–10% of adult AML with an estimated incidence of 0.1/100,000 in Western countries [3]. In the United States, 600–800 new cases are diagnosed every year although the incidence appears increased in patients originating from Latin America [4]. Notably, the median age at diagnosis is approximately 40 years which is significantly lower than in AML where the median age is 68 years.

3.2 Pathogenesis

As mentioned above, the sentinel genetic event behind the pathogenesis of nearly all APL cases is the acquisition of the fusion *PML-RARα* gene. The three most common fusion isoforms are known as the long (bcr1), variant (bcr2), and short (bcr3) isoforms, respectively, and collectively comprise the large majority of *PML-RARα* fusions although other splice variants have been occasionally described [5], and other genetic changes can also yield the same fusion transcripts, in the absence of the canonical t(15;17) [6]. The PML-RARα oncoprotein represses transcription of a number of downstream genes resulting in a maturation arrest at

A. Salhotra (✉) · M. Mei
City of Hope Medical Center, 1500 E Duarte Rd., Duarte, CA 91010, USA
e-mail: asalhotra@coh.org

M. Mei
e-mail: mamei@coh.org

© Springer Nature Switzerland AG 2021
V. Pullarkat and G. Marcucci (eds.), *Biology and Treatment of Leukemia and Bone Marrow Neoplasms*, Cancer Treatment and Research 181,
https://doi.org/10.1007/978-3-030-78311-2_3

the promyelocyte stage. Fusions involving the *RARα* locus and a non-*PML* partner have also been described in APL, the most common of which is *PLZF-RARα* arising from a t(11;17)(q23;q21) [7]. Acquired cytogenetic abnormalities (most commonly trisomy 8) are present in a minority of APL cases and may impact outcomes in patients treated with ATRA and chemotherapy [8]. The somatic mutation landscape has also been characterized and many recurrent mutations have been identified (most commonly in *FLT3*) although in light of the very high cure rate in APL, the impact on prognosis is unclear [9].

3.3 Coagulopathy

Coagulopathy is present in 80% of patients at diagnosis and is a major cause of induction morbidity and mortality. The pathogenesis is complicated and includes significantly increased fibrinolysis, disseminated intravascular coagulopathy, and an increase in inflammatory cytokines [10]. Accordingly, patients typically present with hypofibrinogenemia, thrombocytopenia, and elevated PT/INR and PTT. Mucocutaneous bleeding is fairly common, but more serious intracranial or pulmonary bleeds can also occur [10] and are largely responsible for the significant burden of early death seen in 17–29% patients in the real world setting [11, 12]. Historically, APL was characterized by a rapidly fatal course with a high incidence of early hemorrhagic death. This was evident in early studies when patients who were treated with corticosteroids experienced a median survival of less than 1 week [13, 14]. Early mortality has been significantly reduced by administration of all trans-retinoic acid (ATRA) immediately when the diagnosis is suspected along with aggressive supportive care measures including frequent transfusions of platelets, fresh frozen plasma, and cryoprecipitate while definitive therapy is instituted [15].

3.4 Drug Development in APL

The first therapeutic breakthrough in APL occurred in the 1970s when single-agent daunorubicin was found to induce complete remission (CR) in about 50% of patients with a median duration of response of 26 months [16]. The treatment of APL was further transformed dramatically by the introduction of ATRA and arsenic trioxide (ATO) in 1988 [17] and 1996 [18], respectively. ATRA given at pharmacologic doses binds to the fusion PML-RARα and induces terminal differentiation of APL promyelocytes into mature granulocytes and as monotherapy is associated with CR rates of up to 80% without inducing myelosuppression; however, relapses occur within a few months if no other agents are given [19, 20]. ATO is the single most active agent in APL and was initially tested in the relapsed setting where it was found to induce CR in the large majority of patients [21]. Since then, it has since been incorporated in most of the commonly used frontline regimens as well. It has multiple mechanisms of including both induction of apoptosis and differentiation and potentially via inhibition of angiogenesis as well [22].

3.5 Diagnosis and Initial Management

APL should be suspected in any patient presenting with unexplained DIC and pancytopenia, and the peripheral blood usually shows an excess of promyelocytes. The disease should be treated as a medical emergency given the high early morbidity and mortality, and urgent administration of ATRA should be initiated with aggressive supportive measures including blood product support with platelets to maintain a count of at least 30–50,000/μL and cryoprecipitate to maintain a fibrinogen level of at least 100–150 mg/dL starting even prior to a definitive diagnosis. Leukapheresis is discouraged given that it may exacerbate the coagulopathy [23]. The diagnosis of APL can be quickly confirmed by sending the peripheral blood for *PML-RARα* transcripts by RT-PCR or detecting the PML-RARα fusion gene by fluorescence in situ hybridization (FISH).

3.6 Case 1

JK is a 20-year-old woman who presented with a two-week history of easy bruising and fatigue. A CBC done at presentation showed pancytopenia with a WBC of 1,600/μL, hemoglobin of 8.9 gm/dL and platelet count of 12,000/μL. Coagulation profile showed an elevated INR of 1.4 and a fibrinogen level measuring 58.6 mg/dL. Given the strong suspicion for APL, she was started empirically on ATRA 45 mg/m^2 daily upon arrival to the hospital while further work-up was in progress. FISH testing did reveal a t(15;17), and a bone marrow biopsy revealed 55% blasts positive for CD13, CD33, CD34, CD117, and negative for HLA-DR. She was subsequently started on ATO 0.15 mg/kg IV daily in combination with ATRA 45 mg/m^2. She was monitored closely for differentiation syndrome and during induction therapy, which she tolerated well aside from minor headaches which was treated symptomatically. EKGs were checked 3 times a week to monitor the QT interval and patient received oral calcium, potassium, and magnesium supplementation as needed. A bone marrow biopsy at day 35 showed complete remission, and she subsequently completed 4 cycles of consolidation with ATRA/ATO with the PML-RARα transcript no longer detectable by PCR after the first consolidation cycle. She then received maintenance therapy with ATRA 45 mg/m^2 given for 2 weeks every 3 months for 2 more years. She is now more that 2 years post completion of maintenance therapy and remains in ongoing remission.

3.7 Risk stratification

While APL was previously stratified into low, intermediate, and high-risk disease on the basis of the initial WBC and platelet counts [24], more recently the risk stratification has been simplified and is solely based on the presenting WBC. Patients presenting with an initial WBC measuring $\leq 10,000/\mu L$ are considered to have low-risk disease, and all other patients are considered to have high-risk disease. Of note, while the white count frequently rises after ATRA is initiated due to terminal differentiation of the malignant promyelocytes, the risk stratification is based on the WBC at presentation prior to any therapy.

3.8 Management of Low-Risk Disease

In the pivotal APL0406 study, adult patients with low-risk disease were randomly assigned to either receive ATRA and ATO (ATRA + ATO) for both induction and consolidation or ATRA and idarubicin induction followed by consolidation with ATRA and chemotherapy. The dose of ATRA was 45 mg/m^2 daily, and ATO was given at a dose of 0.15 mg/kg daily. Approximately 75 patients were randomized to each arm with CR rates of 100% and 95% for patients receiving ATRA + ATO and ATRA + chemotherapy, respectively. There were 4 induction deaths in the trial, all of which occurred in patients receiving ATRA + chemotherapy arm. The hematologic toxicity profile was also in favor of using non-chemotherapy induction and maintenance regimen; more differentiation syndrome was seen with ATRA + ATO. 2-year event-free survival rates were 97% and 86%, respectively, in the ATRA + ATO and ATRA + chemotherapy arms [25], and superiority has been confirmed in long-term follow-up [26]. Another multicenter randomized clinical trial conducted in the UK (AML17) compared ATRA plus chemotherapy (idarubicin and mitoxantrone) with ATRA + ATO in adult patients with APL; high-risk patients could receive a dose of the anti-CD33 immunoconjugate gemtuzumab ozogamicin (GO) 6 mg/m^2 on day 1 [27, 28]. The schedule for ATO was slightly different compared to that used in APL0406 with daily dosing for one week followed by twice weekly dosing during induction and consolidation. There was a significantly lower incidence of relapse in patients receiving ATRA + ATO (1 vs. 20% at 5 years) although no difference in OS was seen, likely due to the fact that who had received ATRA + chemotherapy who experienced molecular relapse received ATO salvage. 4-year EFS and OS were 91% and 93%, respectively, in patients receiving ATRA and ATO. On the basis of these two randomized trials, induction therapy combining ATRA + ATO without concurrent cytotoxic chemotherapy is the standard of care for patients with diagnosis of low-risk APL although ATRA + chemotherapy remains an acceptable option when ATO cannot be easily obtained.

3.9 Case 2

BH is a 19-year-old female with no medical history who started to experience mild fatigue and had a cough as well. A CBC was drawn showing a striking leukocytosis with many promyelocytes seen on the smear. She was given a dose of ATRA and urgently transferred to our hospital. On admission, her WBC was 82,000/µL, hemoglobin 8.9 g/dL, and platelet count 97,000/µL; the INR was 1.1 and fibrinogen 120 mg/dL. Urgent FISH testing showed a t(15;17), and a karyotype showed an additional acquired trisomy 8. She was treated according to the APML4 protocol and was given idarubicin 12 mg/m^2 every other day for four doses followed by daily ATO 0.15 mg/kg until remission was achieved; her treatment was complicated by culture-negative neutropenic fever that resolved after count recovery. A bone marrow biopsy after hematologic remission showed no morphologic evidence of residual APL; PCR testing from the aspirate showed that the PML-RARα transcript was still detectable at a level of 9.21×10^{-5}. She then proceeded to two consolidation rounds of ATRA + ATO and two years of maintenance with 6-mercaptopurine, methotrexate, and ATRA. The PML-RARα transcript was no longer molecularly detectable after the first consolidation round, and she remains in ongoing remission, over two years after completion of maintenance therapy.

3.10 High-Risk Disease

Although cytotoxic chemotherapy has been largely eliminated from low-risk treatment regimens, there is less consensus on whether or not to do for patients with high-risk disease given their exclusion from APL0406. The concern with treating high-risk disease with ATRA + ATO alone is that the expected high rate of severe leukocytosis seen with terminal differentiation of the malignant clone; therefore, regimens used for treating high-risk disease have traditionally all included multiple rounds of anthracycline therapy to quickly debulk the disease [29, 30]. Efforts have therefore been focused on reducing the quantity of cytotoxic chemotherapy given or even eliminating it altogether to minimize toxicity. To date, there are two studies which have included high-risk patients while omitting conventional cytotoxic chemotherapy; the results of AML17 were already discussed above, and MD Anderson regimen also incorporated GO (9 mg/m^2 given on day 1) with daily ATRA and ATO with 5-year EFS, DFS, and OS of 81%, 89%, and 86%, respectively [31]. The APML4 trial from the Australasian Leukemia and Lymphoma Group (ALLG) studied ATRA with 4 doses of idarubicin 12 gm/m^2 given every other day followed by daily ATO until remission; no further anthracycline was given. Patients then received two cycles of consolidation therapy with ATRA + ATO followed by 2 years of maintenance therapy with ATRA, 6-mercaptopurine, and methotrexate. 5-year OS and EFS were 94% and 90%, respectively (87 and 83% in the high-risk cohort), and the cumulative incidence of relapse was 5% in high-risk patients [32, 33].

3.11 Practical Aspects of ATRA and ATO Dosing

The recommended starting dose of ATO is 0.15 mg/kg intravenously daily using actual body weight unless the AML17 regimen is utilized. As QT prolongation is one of the principal concerns, regular ECGs are recommended, and every effort should be made to minimize concurrent use of medications that may prolong the QT interval (such as ondansetron and fluoroquinolone antibiotics). Electrolyte levels should be monitored daily, and the potassium and magnesium levels should be maintained at or above 4 mEq/L and 1.8 mg/dL if possible. ATO should be withheld if the QTc exceeds 500 ms until it normalizes; subsequently, it can be resumed afterward at 50% of the dose for a week and gradually escalated back to the full dose. Mild hepatotoxicity in the form of transaminase elevation is also common. In APL0406, ATO was held when the AST and/or ALT exceeded 5 times the upper limit of normal and resumed at 50% of the original dose for a week when they were both under 4 times the upper limit of normal followed by escalation to the full dose. To date, no case of fatal treatment-related hepatotoxicity has been reported in patients treated with ATO. The duration of ATO administered is different depending on the study. For instance, in APL0406 it was given until hematologic remission was achieved or for 60 days, whichever came sooner, whereas AML17 and APML4 both featured fixed durations of ATO (8 weeks for AML17 although it was given 5 days a week for the first week and twice weekly for the subsequent 7 weeks, and 28 consecutive days in APML4).

The recommended starting dose of ATRA is 45 mg/m^2/day given in 2 divided daily doses given until complete remission is achieved. Headache is frequently associated with ATRA use, and if symptomatic management does not alleviate symptoms, the dose may be reduced to 25 mg/m^2/day without impacting efficacy significantly. However, unless there is persistent headache or clearly documented pseudotumor cerebri, dose reduction is not recommended. Additionally, patients receiving ATRA should be closely monitored for hyperleukocytosis (only during induction), differentiation syndrome (discussed below), and liver function abnormalities.

3.12 Differentiation Syndrome

Differentiation syndrome is a potentially life-threatening complication which can occur within the first few days to weeks after the start of ATRA and/or ATO-based induction and is associated with one or more of the following clinical manifestations: dyspnea, pulmonary interstitial infiltrates, fever, weight gain, pleuropericardial effusions, hypotension, acute renal failure, and peripheral edema. It is thought to be mediated at least in part by massive cytokine release from the maturing precursor myeloid cells [34]. As these findings may also be associated with infection or hemorrhage, differentiation syndrome is a diagnosis of exclusion [35]. Careful attention to supportive care and prompt initiation of glucocorticoids (typically dexamethasone 10 mg IV twice daily) is imperative. In mild to moderate cases, continuation of ATRA and/or ATO is reasonable; in severe cases, holding these agents and resuming after there is clinical improvement is recommended [36]. Of note, some regimens including APL0406 and APML4 include prophylactic corticosteroids.

3.13 Pseudotumor Cerebri (PTC)

This is a rare complication of ATRA therapy with a reported incidence of 3% in randomized studies [23]. It is seen mainly in children and adolescents and characterized by headache and evidence of papilledema on ophthalmologic examination. Neuroimaging is required for exclusion of intracranial space-occupying lesions and spinal fluid analysis is also required. Management is by temporary discontinuation of ATRA if symptoms persist after use of analgesic medications. Acetazolamide and steroids can also help alleviate the symptoms.

3.14 Response Assessment and Surveillance

The large majority of patients who receive ATRA plus chemotherapy or ATRA plus ATO achieve remission at the end of induction chemotherapy unless they succumb to early infectious or hemorrhagic complications. During the first 3–4 weeks of induction therapy, the white count frequently rises which signifies terminal differentiation of the malignant clone and indicates neither marrow recovery nor progressive disease. Treatment should continue until there is no morphologic evidence of disease in the bone marrow, and in our experience patients often require 5–6 weeks to achieve morphologic remission with full count recovery. Of note, most patients will still have molecularly detectable disease after induction therapy, and there is no need to test for the *PML-RARα* until the end of consolidation. The ultimate goal of treatment is to achieve a complete molecular remission defined as an undetectable *PML-RARα* transcript level in the bone marrow by RT-PCR [37, 38].

As relapse is relatively uncommon for patients who are treated with ATRA and ATO containing regimens, there is no standard of post-treatment surveillance for patients who achieve molecular remission. The role of surveillance in low-risk patients treated with ATRA and ATO is unclear given the low risk of relapse. In high-risk patients where the rate of relapse is higher and exceeds 10%, surveillance PCR from the peripheral blood every 2–3 months for 2 years after the completion of consolidation and/or maintenance is reasonable as either a molecular or overt relapse warrants salvage therapy as outlined below.

3.15 Role of Maintenance Therapy

Although many older APL regimens include an extended period of maintenance therapy, its efficacy is unclear in low-risk patients treated with ATRA and ATO as well as in high-risk patients whose frontline therapy include both ATRA and ATO. The APL93 trial whose induction and consolidation therapy both consisted of ATRA, daunorubicin, and cytarabine found a decreased 10-year relapse rate with 2 years of maintenance ATRA, 6-mercaptopurine, and methotrexate [39]. The North American APL Intergroup Study found benefit to maintenance ATRA therapy although the induction and consolidation regimens are inferior to those presently used (induction and the first consolidation were both randomized to ATRA vs. daunorubicin and cytarabine) [40]. Also, APML4 included maintenance therapy with ATRA, 6-mercaptopurine, and methotrexate in all patients. However, neither APL0406 and AML17 included maintenance therapy. For any given patient, we recommend full adherence to the regimen as published with implementation of maintenance if it is part of the chosen regimen.

3.16 Case 3

MT is a 40-year-old woman who presented to outside hospital with heavy menstrual bleeding, headaches, and easy bruising. A CBC was significant for a WBC count of 15,000/μL, platelet count of 20,000/μL, and hemoglobin of 8.8 gm/dL. The INR was 1.4 and fibrinogen was 110 mg/dL at presentation. Bone marrow biopsy confirmed APL with a hypercellular marrow showing 70% promyelocytes, and a karyotype showed 46 XX, t(15;17)(q24;q21). She received induction chemotherapy with ATRA, ATO, and 4 doses of idarubicin at 12 mg/m^2 given on days 2, 4, 6, and 8 due to her high-risk disease; induction was complicated by headaches requiring dose reduction in ATRA. A bone marrow biopsy was done 6 weeks post induction chemotherapy confirmed that the patient had received morphologic and cytogenetic remission. She then completed 4 cycles of ATRA + ATO consolidation. She presented one year later with similar symptoms, and a bone marrow biopsy confirmed relapsed APL. She achieved molecular remission with ATRA + ATO and underwent autologous hematopoietic cell transplant (ASCT) conditioned with fractionated total body irradiation and etoposide. At 6 months post ASCT, she remains in molecular remission.

3.17 Management of Relapsed APL

With introduction of ATRA and ATO alone in low-risk patients and the increasing use of ATRA and ATO with a third agent in high-risk disease, the large majority of patients will achieve long term cure provided the full course of therapy is delivered.

However, a fraction of patients still relapse and need salvage therapy. In the event of an early relapse occurring within 6 months f completion of ATRA and ATO-based therapy without prior anthracycline, ATRA + anthracycline therapy is reasonable. In the event of a later relapse (over 6 months) or early relapse after ATRA + chemotherapy, ATO therapy is recommended with an unclear benefit for the addition of ATRA. If molecular remission is achieved, then autologous transplant is recommended with curative intent and appears to be superior to allogeneic transplant when performed in second remission [41].

References

1. Wang ZY, Chen Z (2008) Acute promyelocytic leukemia: from highly fatal to highly curable. Blood 111(5):2505–2515
2. Lallemand-Breitenbach V, Guillemin MC, Janin A et al (1999) Retinoic acid and arsenic synergize to eradicate leukemic cells in a mouse model of acute promyelocytic leukemia. J Exp Med 189(7):1043–1052
3. Sant M, Allemani C, Tereanu C et al (2010) Incidence of hematologic malignancies in Europe by morphologic subtype: results of the HAEMACARE project. Blood 116(19):3724–3734
4. Douer D (2003) The epidemiology of acute promyelocytic leukaemia. Best Pract Res Clin Haematol 16(3):357–367
5. Pandolfi PP, Alcalay M, Fagioli M et al (1992) Genomic variability and alternative splicing generate multiple PML/RAR alpha transcripts that encode aberrant PML proteins and PML/RAR alpha isoforms in acute promyelocytic leukaemia. EMBO J 11(4):1397–1407
6. Grimwade D, Biondi A, Mozziconacci MJ et al (2000) Characterization of acute promyelocytic leukemia cases lacking the classic t(15;17): results of the European Working Party. Groupe Francais de Cytogenetique Hematologique, Groupe de Francais d'Hematologie Cellulaire, UK Cancer Cytogenetics Group and BIOMED 1 European Community-Concerted Action "Molecular Cytogenetic Diagnosis in Haematological Malignancies". Blood 96 (4):1297–1308
7. Redner RL (2002) Variations on a theme: the alternate translocations in APL. Leukemia 16 (10):1927–1932
8. Cervera J, Montesinos P, Hernández-Rivas JM et al (2010) Additional chromosome abnormalities in patients with acute promyelocytic leukemia treated with all-trans retinoic acid and chemotherapy. Haematologica 95(3):424–431
9. Awada H, Durrani J, Kewan TZ, Kishtagari A, Visconte V, Mahfouz RZ (2019) Comprehensive characterization of cytogenetic and mutational analysis of acute promyelocytic Leukemia: is PML-Rara everything? Blood 134(Supplement_1):1404–1404
10. Breen KA, Grimwade D, Hunt BJ (2012) The pathogenesis and management of the coagulopathy of acute promyelocytic leukaemia. Br J Haematol 156(1):24–36
11. McClellan JS, Kohrt HE, Coutre S et al (2012) Treatment advances have not improved the early death rate in acute promyelocytic leukemia. Haematologica 97(1):133–136
12. Park JH, Qiao B, Panageas KS et al (2011) Early death rate in acute promyelocytic leukemia remains high despite all-trans retinoic acid. Blood 118(5):1248–1254
13. Pisciotta AV, Schulz EJ (1955) Fibrinolytic purpura in acute leukemia. Am J Med 19 (5):824–828
14. Cooperberg AA, Neiman GM (1955) Fibrinogenopenia and fibrinolysis in acute myelogenous leukemia. Ann Intern Med 42(3):706–711
15. Seftel MD, Barnett MJ, Couban S et al (2014) A Canadian consensus on the management of newly diagnosed and relapsed acute promyelocytic leukemia in adults. Curr Oncol (Toronto, Ont) 21(5):234–250

16. Bernard J, Weil M, Boiron M, Jacquillat C, Flandrin G, Gemon M-F (1973) Acute promyelocytic leukemia: results of treatment by daunorubicin. Blood 41(4):489–496; (2016) Blood 128(14):1779

17. Huang ME, Ye YC, Chen SR et al (1988) Use of all-trans retinoic acid in the treatment of acute promyelocytic leukemia. Blood 72(2):567–572; (2016) Blood 128(26):3017

18. Chen GQ, Zhu J, Shi XG et al (1996) In vitro studies on cellular and molecular mechanisms of arsenic trioxide (As_2O_3) in the treatment of acute promyelocytic leukemia: As_2O_3 induces NB4 cell apoptosis with downregulation of Bcl-2 expression and modulation of PML-RAR alpha/PML proteins. Blood 88(3):1052–1061

19. Warrell RP Jr, Frankel SR, Miller WH Jr et al (1991) Differentiation therapy of acute promyelocytic leukemia with tretinoin (all-trans-retinoic acid). N Engl J Med 324 (20):1385–1393

20. Sanz MA, Lo-Coco F (2011) Modern approaches to treating acute promyelocytic leukemia. J Clin Oncol: Official J Am Soc Clin Oncol 29(5):495–503

21. Lengfelder E, Hofmann WK, Nowak D (2012) Impact of arsenic trioxide in the treatment of acute promyelocytic leukemia. Leukemia 26(3):433–442

22. Falchi L, Verstovsek S, Ravandi-Kashani F, Kantarjian HM (2016) The evolution of arsenic in the treatment of acute promyelocytic leukemia and other myeloid neoplasms: moving toward an effective oral, outpatient therapy. Cancer 122(8):1160–1168

23. Sanz MA, Grimwade D, Tallman MS et al (2009) Management of acute promyelocytic leukemia: recommendations from an expert panel on behalf of the European LeukemiaNet. Blood 113(9):1875–1891

24. Sanz MA, Lo Coco F, Martin G et al (2000) Definition of relapse risk and role of nonanthracycline drugs for consolidation in patients with acute promyelocytic leukemia: a joint study of the PETHEMA and GIMEMA cooperative groups. Blood 96(4):1247–1253

25. Lo-Coco F, Avvisati G, Vignetti M et al (2013) Retinoic acid and arsenic trioxide for acute promyelocytic leukemia. N Engl J Med 369(2):111–121

26. Cicconi L, Platzbecker U, Avvisati G et al (2019) Long-term results of all-trans retinoic acid and arsenic trioxide in non-high-risk acute promyelocytic leukemia: update of the APL0406 Italian-German randomized trial. Leukemia

27. Russell N, Burnett A, Hills R et al (2018) Attenuated arsenic trioxide plus ATRA therapy for newly diagnosed and relapsed APL: long-term follow-up of the AML17 trial. Blood 132 (13):1452–1454

28. Burnett AK, Russell NH, Hills RK et al (2015) Arsenic trioxide and all-trans retinoic acid treatment for acute promyelocytic leukaemia in all risk groups (AML17): results of a randomised, controlled, phase 3 trial. The Lancet. Oncol 16(13):1295–1305

29. Lo-Coco F, Avvisati G, Vignetti M et al (2010) Front-line treatment of acute promyelocytic leukemia with AIDA induction followed by risk-adapted consolidation for adults younger than 61 years: results of the AIDA-2000 trial of the GIMEMA Group. Blood 116 (17):3171–3179

30. Powell BL, Moser B, Stock W et al (2010) Arsenic trioxide improves event-free and overall survival for adults with acute promyelocytic leukemia: North American Leukemia Intergroup Study C9710. Blood 116(19):3751–3757

31. Abaza Y, Kantarjian H, Garcia-Manero G et al (2017) Long-term outcome of acute promyelocytic leukemia treated with all-trans-retinoic acid, arsenic trioxide, and gemtuzumab. Blood 129(10):1275–1283

32. Iland HJ, Collins M, Bradstock K et al (2015) Use of arsenic trioxide in remission induction and consolidation therapy for acute promyelocytic leukaemia in the Australasian Leukaemia and Lymphoma Group (ALLG) APML4 study: a non-randomised phase 2 trial. The Lancet. Haematol 2(9):e357–366

33. Iland HJ, Bradstock K, Supple SG et al (2012) All-trans-retinoic acid, idarubicin, and IV arsenic trioxide as initial therapy in acute promyelocytic leukemia (APML4). Blood 120 (8):1570–1580; quiz 1752

34. Luesink M, Jansen JH (2010) Advances in understanding the pulmonary infiltration in acute promyelocytic leukaemia. Br J Haematol 151(3):209–220
35. Frankel SR, Eardley A, Lauwers G, Weiss M, Warrell RP Jr (1992) The "retinoic acid syndrome" in acute promyelocytic leukemia. Ann Intern Med 117(4):292–296
36. Sanz MA, Montesinos P (2014) How we prevent and treat differentiation syndrome in patients with acute promyelocytic leukemia. Blood 123(18):2777–2782
37. Lo Coco F, Diverio D, Falini B, Biondi A, Nervi C, Pelicci PG (1999) Genetic diagnosis and molecular monitoring in the management of acute promyelocytic leukemia. Blood 94 (1):12–22
38. Grimwade D, Lo CF (2002) Acute promyelocytic leukemia: a model for the role of molecular diagnosis and residual disease monitoring in directing treatment approach in acute myeloid leukemia. Leukemia 16(10):1959–1973
39. Ades L, Guerci A, Raffoux E et al (2010) Very long-term outcome of acute promyelocytic leukemia after treatment with all-trans retinoic acid and chemotherapy: the European APL Group experience. Blood 115(9):1690–1696
40. Tallman MS, Andersen JW, Schiffer CA et al (2002) All-trans retinoic acid in acute promyelocytic leukemia: long-term outcome and prognostic factor analysis from the North American Intergroup protocol. Blood 100(13):4298–4302
41. Holter Chakrabarty JL, Rubinger M, Le-Rademacher J et al (2014) Autologous is superior to allogeneic hematopoietic cell transplantation for acute promyelocytic leukemia in second complete remission. Biol Blood Marrow Trans 20(7):1021–1025

Current and Emerging Therapies for Acute Myeloid Leukemia

4

Brian Ball, Matthew Mei, Salman Otoukesh, and Anthony Stein

Contents

B. Ball (✉) · M. Mei · S. Otoukesh · A. Stein
City of Hope Medical Center, 1500 E Duarte Rd., Duarte, CA 91010, USA
e-mail: brball@coh.org

M. Mei
e-mail: mamei@coh.org

S. Otoukesh
e-mail: sotoukesh@coh.org

A. Stein
e-mail: AStein@coh.org

© Springer Nature Switzerland AG 2021
V. Pullarkat and G. Marcucci (eds.), *Biology and Treatment of Leukemia and Bone Marrow Neoplasms*, Cancer Treatment and Research 181,
https://doi.org/10.1007/978-3-030-78311-2_4

4.1 Introduction

Acute myeloid leukemia (AML) is characterized by blocked differentiation and proliferation of immature myeloid cells leading to bone marrow failure and infiltration of other organs. Although significant advances in therapy have been realized in recent years, overall outcomes remain poor, especially in elderly and unfit patients who comprise the majority of AML patients. In fit patients, induction therapy has historically consisted of a combination of an anthracycline such as idarubicin or daunorubicin and infusional cytarabine with the goal of achieving a morphologic complete remission (CR) defined by recovery of normal hematopoiesis and less than 5% myeloid blasts in the bone marrow. However, even if a CR is realized, relapse is inevitable without further consolidation therapy, either with additional cycles of cytotoxic chemotherapy or with allogeneic stem cell transplantation (alloSCT), with the specific decision regarding consolidation therapy dependent on the probability of relapse based on cytogenetics and molecular studies. Most patients who achieve CR are consolidated with alloSCT with curative intent if they are suitable candidates with available donors. Elderly or unfit patients were traditionally treated with hypomethylating agents alone or offered the best supportive care. Lately, a combination of hypomethylating agent with the Bcl-2 inhibitor venetoclax has shown marked efficacy in AML and has become the standard of care for the elderly and unfit patient population. This has allowed more patients in the older age groups to achieve deep CR and proceed to alloSCT using reduced-intensity conditioning. For patients with relapsed or refractory (R/R) disease, outcomes remain poor and for the majority of cases without a targetable mutation, there is no standard treatment regimen. Choice of therapy in R/R AML is based on several factors such as patient fitness, alloSCT candidacy, and molecular profiling with the ultimate goal of doing alloSCT, ideally performed while in second complete remission.

While the above outline still holds true, a deep understanding of the molecular biology underpinning AML continues to be translated into therapeutic advances, many of which are rapidly being incorporated into standard practice. In particular, a number of targeted therapies directed at individual driver mutations have been approved in AML, both as single agents as well as in conjunction with cytotoxic chemotherapy, and play an important role in the current management of AML. Moreover, the development of antibody-based therapies, T-cell-based immunotherapy, and additional apoptosis-inducing therapies is accelerating as well and it is highly likely that these approaches will also take their place in the hematologist's armamentarium in the near future. In this chapter, we will summarize current as well as emerging therapeutic approaches in AML.

4.1.1 Case 1

A 73-year-old previously healthy male presented with fatigue and was noted to have a white blood count of 33,000/μL hemoglobin of 7.9g/dL, and platelet count of 56,000/μL.

A bone marrow biopsy showed normal karyotype AML, and limited molecular testing done was significant for a wild-type FLT3 and the presence of a 4-bp insertion in the NPM1 gene. He was induced with daunorubicin 60 mg/m^2 for 3 days and cytarabine 200 mg/m^2 for 7 days and achieved complete remission and was subsequently consolidated with three cycles of high-dose cytarabine dosed at 2 gm/m^2 for 6 doses in each cycle, the last of which was complicated by a perirectal abscess requiring incision and drainage.

4.2 Induction Therapy

Induction therapy in AML for fit patients has traditionally consisted of three daily doses of an anthracycline (typically either daunorubicin or idarubicin) in conjunction with infusional cytarabine given for 7 days, a combination that is commonly termed 7 + 3. Either daunorubicin or idarubicin can be given, and while earlier data suggested improved clinical efficacy with a daunorubicin dose of 90 mg/m^2 as opposed to 45 or 60 mg/m^2, a more recent randomized trial showed that there was no benefit in the 90 mg/m^2 dose versus 60 mg/m^2 except potentially in the subgroup of patients whose disease harbored a FLT3-ITD abnormality [1, 2]. With this approach, CR rates are in the 70% range but vary according to molecular and cytogenetic risk stratification. This approach is, however, associated with significant toxicity with prolonged periods of pancytopenia being the rule, and the risk of early mortality approaches 10% [3]. Of note, the definition of fitness is a subjective one and incorporates age, performance status, and other medical comorbidities, especially cardiac comorbidities that would potentially be prohibitive for anthracycline administration, but is ultimately at the discretion of the treating physician [4].

Other variations of intensive induction built on the backbone of 7 + 3 exist as well; 7 + 3 in conjunction with five daily doses of cladribine 5 mg/m^2 was studied in a randomized trial against 7 + 3 by Holowiecki et al. and found to associated with a higher CR rate and increased OS; however, this trial was criticized for an abnormally low CR rate in the control arm (56%) and lack of an early bone marrow aspirate 1-week post-induction to help guide the decision for the second round of induction therapy [5]. The CD33-directed antibody–drug conjugate (ADC) gemtuzumab ozogamicin (GO, Mylotarg ®) was approved for adults with newly diagnosed CD33-expressing AML on the basis of the ALFA-0701 trial combining administration of GO 3 mg/m^2 on days 1, 4, and 7 with 7 + 3. -Two year event-free survival was improved with the administration of GO (40.8 vs. 17.1%), although there was not a statistically significant improvement in OS [6]. A large meta-analysis of 3325 patients who received GO with induction therapy showed an improved OS at 5 years and suggested that patients with favorable risk cytogenetics derived the most benefit, but patients with intermediate-risk cytogenetic abnormalities also enjoyed improved OS as well while patients with adverse cytogenetics did not benefit [7]. Of note, 5% of patients receiving GO in ALFA-0701 subsequently developed veno-occlusive disease [6], an important consideration in patients for whom alloSCT is being contemplated. Finally, the addition of the small molecular tyrosine kinase inhibitor midostaurin (Rydapt®) on days 8–21 after standard induction and consolidation is approved for patients with newly diagnosed AML which harbors either a FLT3 internal tandem duplication (FLT3-ITD) or FLT3-tyrosine kinase domain (FLT3-TKD) mutation on the basis of a randomized phase 3 trial that showed improvement in both EFS and OS seen with the addition of midostaurin (Rydapt®) [8].

Apart from 7 + 3, CPX-351 (Vyxeos ®), a liposomal formulation of cytarabine and daunorubicin in a fixed 5:1 ratio, was approved as a single agent for induction therapy of AML in adults older than 60 years with high risk or secondary AML on the basis of an open-label randomized trial where it was evaluated against 7 + 3.[9] High risk or secondary AML was specifically defined as therapy-related AML and AML with myelodysplastic related changes (AML with antecedent myelodysplastic syndrome (MDS), AML with 50% or more dysplastic cells in at least two cell lines, and AML with MDS-related cytogenetic abnormalities). The median OS and CR rate were higher with CPX-351 as opposed to 7 + 3, while early mortality and overall safety were comparable despite more protracted count recovery with CPX-351. Furthermore, CPX-351 appears to be an effective bridge to subsequent alloSCT as well [10].

For the patient presented in Case 1 above, the decision was made by the treating physician to administer 7 + 3 based on his excellent performance status and favorable risk profile (normal cytogenetics with wild type FLT3 status and mutated NPM1) despite his advanced age in order to give him the benefit of potentially curative therapy. However, it must be mentioned that in actual clinical practice the vast majority of patients at his age would not be candidates for intensive chemotherapy by virtue of comorbidities as well as adverse leukemia genetics and would be best served by lower intensity approaches discussed below.

4.2.1 Induction Therapy for Unfit Patients

For the unfit patient, although a number of options in the frontline setting still existed, until recently the available options yielded low response rates. Although these patients are generally incurable, a hypomethylating agent (HMA) such as decitabine or 5-azacytidine or low-dose chemotherapy were the treatments that were commonly used. Single-agent decitabine given for a 5-day course at 20 mg/m^2 every 28 days compared to physician's choice of low-dose cytarabine or supportive care was associated with a trend towards improved OS on the primary analysis with similar safety; notably, the CR/CRp rate was 18.8% with decitabine [11]. A 10-day course of decitabine at the same dose of 20 mg/m^2 appears to be associated with higher response rates albeit not in a randomized trial [12] and seems to be particularly effective in patients whose AML harbors a TP53 mutation [13]. Another treatment option includes single-agent GO, which showed a very modest OS advantage of 1.3 months compared to best supportive care in elderly patients in the EORTC-GIMEMA AML19 trial [14]. Additionally, the hedgehog inhibitor, glasdegib in combination with low dose cytarabine is approved for elderly patients (age $\geq$ 75 years) with newly diagnosed AML unsuitable for intensive chemotherapy based on the phase 2 BRIGHT AML 1003 trial, which demonstrated higher response rates (CR/CRi rate: 17 vs. 2%, $p < 0.05$) and prolonged survival (median OS: 8.8 vs. 4.9 months, $p = 0.0004$) with the combination when compared to low-dose cytarabine alone [15].

More recently, the outlook for the frail, older, and unfit patients has markedly improved with the approval of HMA in combination with venetoclax for this population. The combination of HMA with venetoclax, an orally bioavailable, selective BCL-2 inhibitor, has been found to be very active for newly diagnosed AML in elderly and unfit patients with a CR/CRi rate of 67% and a median duration of response of 11.3 months. Moreover, the results showed CR/CRi of 60% and 65% in poor cytogenetics and elderly (>75 yrs old), respectively [16]. The combination of HMA with venetoclax is well tolerated and lacks significant organ toxicity except for the major side effect of cytopenia. Venetoclax dosing requires adjustment when given concomitantly with CYP3A4-inhibiting antifungals (e.g., posaconazole and voriconazole) [17]. The combination of low dose Ara-C and venetoclax similarly demonstrated a high rates CR/CRi of 54% with a median survival of 10.1 months in a phase 1/2 trial of untreated patients 60 years or older ineligible for intensive chemotherapy [18]. Although both regimens are approved for the treatment of newly diagnosed AML for patients over 75 years of age or unfit for conventional induction chemotherapy, only venetoclax in combination with HMA led to significantly longer survival in phase 3 trials and is considered the preferred regimen for previously untreated patients unfit for intensive chemotherapy [19, 20].

4.3 Post-Remission Consolidation

Post-remission therapy of AML typically consists of either consolidation chemotherapy or allogeneic stem cell transplantation (alloSCT). In general, alloSCT reduces the rate of relapse but at the cost of increased toxicity and treatment-related mortality. Patients with favorable risk disease by the 2017 European Leukemia Net guidelines generally do not proceed to alloSCT, while in the first CR given the significant curative potential of consolidation chemotherapy alone [21], while strong consideration should be made for consolidative alloSCT in all other patients who are physically fit and have a donor [22]. High-dose cytarabine (HIDAC) is the most common consolidation regimen and is usually given for 3–4 cycles; a cytarabine dose of 3 gm/m^2 twice daily on days 1, 3, and 5 was shown to be superior to cytarabine dosed at 100 and 400 mg/m^2 for five consecutive days [23], and patients over 60 typically receive a dose reduction to 2 gm/m^2 due to significant toxicity. If alloSCT is to be considered and a donor is available, it should be done without delay as there does not appear to be any benefit derived from further consolidation chemotherapy with HIDAC after achieving an initial remission [24, 25]. There may be an advantage to myeloablative conditioning in patients who are able to tolerate a more intense approach [26]. The use of HMA with venetoclax by virtue of its quick response and high CR rate would be expected to permit more older patients, particularly in the 60–75 age range to undergo potential curative reduced-intensity alloSCT.

4.3.1 Case 1 (Continued)

Approximately 18 months after his final cycle of consolidation with high-dose cytarabine, he developed pancytopenia, and a bone marrow biopsy confirmed relapsed AML. Comprehensive molecular testing now showed a persistent NPM1 mutation without a concomitant FLT3 abnormality, but an IDH1 R132H mutation was also identified; IDH1 and IDH2 mutation testing was not performed at the time of his initial diagnosis. He was treated with the oral IDH1 inhibitor ivosidenib (AG-120) as monotherapy on a clinical protocol. One month after commencing therapy, he remained with 14% circulating blasts and a bone marrow biopsy showed 35% blasts, but he cleared his peripheral blasts in the subsequent month, and a bone marrow biopsy performed after 2 months of therapy confirmed complete remission with persistent mild pancytopenia, and he had full count recovery one month later.

4.4 Relapsed/Refractory Disease

With the rapid development of targeted therapies, there are more options available for such patients besides salvage with conventional cytotoxic chemotherapy which is associated with low response rates and significant toxicity. However, any final therapeutic decision must take into account the patient's clinical status (i.e., age, performance status, transplant candidacy, duration of first remission) as well as the disease biology and in particular the presence or absence of actionable mutations. In general, for r/r AML the only potentially curative option is alloSCT, ideally performed after morphologic remission is achieved.

A number of intensive reinduction regimens with cytotoxic chemotherapy have been used in r/r AML including fludarabine, cytarabine, G-CSF (FLAG), mitoxantrone, etoposide, and cytarabine (MEC), and high-dose cytarabine (HIDAC) [27–29]. There are no data to specifically recommend one over another, and toxicity is significant. As these regimens are not curative without subsequent alloSCT, the general goal of intensive reinduction is to serve as a bridge for the fit patient to undergo alloSCT.

Approximately 20% of patients with AML will have a mutation in either *isocitrate dehydrogenase-1 (IDH1)* or *isocitrate dehydrogenase-2 (IDH2)*. These mutations result in an aberrant reduction of alpha-ketoglutarate to 2-hydroxyglutarate, the latter being an abnormal oncometabolite that leads to abnormal DNA methylation [30]. The IDH2 inhibitor enasidenib (Idhifa®) was approved in 2017 as single-agent therapy for patients with *IDH2*-mutated AML on the basis of a phase 1/2 trial showing an overall response rate (ORR) of 40% and median response duration of 5.8 months and OS of 9.3 months; the CR rate was 19.3% and in patients who achieved CR, OS was 19.7 months. 44% of patients experienced a grade 3–4 treatment-related adverse events, most commonly hyperbilirubinemia (12%), hematologic adverse events (10%), and differentiation syndrome (6%) [31]. Subsequently, the IDH1 inhibitor ivosidenib (Tibsovo®) was approved in 2018 for patients with *IDH1*-mutated AML on the basis of a phase 1 trial of 258 patients; ORR was 41.6%, median response duration was 8.2 months, and overall survival was 8.8 months. Among the patients who achieved CR, slightly more than half were alive at 18 months (50.1%). Among them, 20.7% of patients had a grade 3–4 treatment-related adverse events, most commonly QT interval prolongation (7.8%) and differentiation syndrome (3.9%) [32]. At present, there are no published randomized data comparing IDH1 or IDH2 inhibitors to conventional chemotherapy, and the decision of optimal therapy for the patient with r/r AML carrying an *IDH1* or *IDH2* mutation must take into account physical fitness, candidacy for allo-HCT, and prior response to induction chemotherapy.

Finally, hypomethylating agents alone have been used in the r/r setting, but data have primarily been in the form of single-center retrospective studies. Results from a larger multicenter retrospective study of 655 patients were recently reported with a CR/CRi rate of 16.3% and median OS of 6.7 months; patients achieving a CR/CRi had a median OS of 21 months. A higher blast percentage portended worse survival, but there was no clear association of cytogenetics, WBC at relapse, or age with clinical outcomes [33].

4.4.1 Case 1 (Continued)

He relapsed again 16 months after starting the AG-120 and was then treated with decitabine 20 mg/m^2 for 5 consecutive days in conjunction with venetoclax 400 mg p.o. daily. He developed neutropenic fever shortly after starting therapy, but he then recovered his counts rapidly and was found to be in remission after his first cycle. He continues to be treated with decitabine and venetoclax every 28 days and remains in remission at this time, 5 months after starting this therapy.

4.5 FLT3-Mutated AML

4.5.1 Case 2

A 70-year-old male with a history of treated colon and renal cancer was found having a white blood count of 27000/μL, hemoglobin of 8.1 g/dL, and platelet of 146,000/μL. A bone marrow biopsy showed AML with monocytic differentiation, cytogenetic analysis showed 46,XY,t(10;11), and molecular testing revealed FLT3-ITD. He was induced with idarubicin and cytarabine (7+3) in combination with midostaurin on days 8–21. Induction was complicated by neutropenic fever.

The cytokine receptor tyrosine kinase, *FMS-like tyrosine kinase 3 (FLT3)* is the most commonly mutated gene in AML, occurring in approximately 30% of newly diagnosed patients younger than 65 years [34]. Activating mutations of the *FLT3* gene occur as in-frame internal tandem duplications (ITD) of between 3 and more than 100 amino acids located in the juxtamembrane region or as missense point mutations in the tyrosine kinase domain (TKD). Of the two classes of mutations, FLT3 internal tandem duplications (ITD) are more troublesome, being associated with an increased risk of relapse and subsequently death after transplantation [35, 36]. An elevated white blood cell count at diagnosis is characteristic of *FLT3-ITD* mutant AML and $\sim 30\%$ of patients presenting with hyperleukocytosis (WBC > 50 $\times$ 10^9/L) harbor the abnormality [37]. The mutation burden or allelic ratio of mutant *FLT3-ITD* to wild type correlates with disease burden and an allelic ratio > 0.5 increases relapse risk after transplantation [21, 38, 39]. Additionally, longer FLT3-ITD duplications confer resistance to chemotherapy and decreased survival [38, 40, 41]. Over the past 20 years, significant strides have been in the development of effective FLT3 targeting therapy. First-generation inhibitors, such as midostaurin, lestaurtinib, and sunitnib are less selective, inhibiting FLT3 as well as many other kinases, and have demonstrated modest efficacy in clinical studies [42–44]. However, combinations of FLT3 inhibitors with chemotherapy have the potential to induce deeper remissions than induction chemotherapy alone. In the seminal phase 3 RATIFY study, patients randomized to treatment with the addition of the multitargeted kinase inhibitor, midostaurin to standard induction and consolidation chemotherapy and maintenance had significantly longer median survival (74.7 months vs. 25.6 months, HR = 0.78, $p = 0.009$) and event-free survival (8.2 months vs. 3 months, HR 0.78, $p = 0.002$) when compared to patients treated with placebo [8]. A subsequent phase 2 study by the German-Austrian AML Study Group (AMLSG 16–10) showed that midostaurin maintenance prolonged event-free survival in all groups (transplant and non-transplant) as well as in the elderly population [45].

4.5.2   Case 2 (Continued)

Bone marrow biopsy on day28 after initiation of chemotherapy showed persistent disease with 14% myeloid blasts in the marrow and molecular testing again revealed *FLT3-ITD* mutation. He was treated with gilteritinib and had a partial response with a decrease in bone marrow blasts to 6% which lasted for 2 months. The patient subsequently developed progression of his disease and acheived a CR after treatment with HMA +Venetoclax.

After progression on intensive induction chemotherapy and midostaurin, patients remain eligible for other FLT3 targeting therapy. Second-generation inhibitors, including gilteritinib, crenolanib, and quizartinib are more selective and potent inhibitors of FLT3. FLT3 inhibitors are further classified by the site of binding on the FLT3 protein. Whereas type 1 inhibitors (e.g., midostaurin, gilteritinib, and crenolanib) bind to the ATP binding site in the active pocket of the enzyme, type II inhibitors (e.g., sorafenib and quizartinib) bind to a hydrophobic pocket adjacent to the ATP-binding site when the protein is in its inactive conformation [34, 46]. The distinction is relevant because activating mutations in the FLT3 kinase domain or gatekeeper residue lock the protein in an active confirmation or directly disrupt the hydrophobic binding site to confer resistance to type II inhibitors [34, 47, 48]. As a result, the type II inhibitor, quizartinib induces responses primarily in patients with FLT3-ITD mutations rather than FLT3 TKD-mutated patients. In a phase 3 study, patients with R/R AML with *FLT3-ITD* mutations randomized to quizartinib had longer survival (median OS: 6.2 months vs. 4.7 months, $p = 0.02$) and were more likely to proceed to alloSCT (32 vs. 11%), when compared to patients receiving salvage chemotherapy [49]. However, treatment with quizartinib is limited by the frequent emergence of resistance-conferring FLT3 TKD mutations at the time of relapse [48]. Crenolanib is a promising pan FLT3 (ITD and TKD) inhibitor that led to responses in 47% and a median survival of 19 weeks for patients with R/R AML with FLT3 ITD or TKD mutations in a phase 2 study and phase 3 studies are ongoing. **Gilteritinib** is an oral highly potent pan-FLT3 inhibitor and the only FLT3 inhibitor currently approved for patients with R/R AML harboring *FLT3* mutations. Approval was based on the seminal phase 3 ADMIRAL trial, which demonstrated higher complete remission rates with full or partial hematologic recovery (34 vs. 15%), prolonged survival (median OS: 9.3 months vs. 5.6 months, $p < 0.001$), and a higher rate of alloSCT (26 vs. 15%) among patients with *FLT3*-mutated R/R AML randomized to gilteritinib when compared to salvage chemotherapy. However, most patients responding to the type I inhibitors, gilteritinib, and crenolanib inevitably relapse with resistance most frequently arising due to the acquisition of *RAS* signaling pathway mutations [50, 51].

The combination of venetoclax with hypomethylating agents or low-dose cytarabine also has demonstrated activity in the relapsed or refractory setting and is currently the regimen of choice in many patients regardless of mutation status. Complete remissions when achieved occur quickly, mostly after 1 cycle and could allow more patients to proceed to potentially curative alloSCT. The excellent tolerability of this regimen, lack of organ toxicity are added advantages, particularly in alloSCT candidates. Evidence of efficacy is limited to mostly retrospective studies, however, a meta-analysis of seven studies demonstrated a composite ORR of 39% and CR/CRi rate of 33% for venetoclax combinations [52]. Despite many patients achieving a deep and durable remission with venetoclax-based regimens, primary and secondary resistance is known to occur through the acquisition of *FLT3*, *RAS*, or *TP53* mutations as well as other mechanisms [53]. In contrast, the presence of *NPM1* or *IDH* mutations is associated with increased responses to venetoclax regimens [53].

4.6 Other Novel Targeted Therapies

Menin Inhibitors (SNDX-5613 and MI-3454) Rearrangement of the *lysine methyltransferase 2A (KMT2A)* gene, previously known as *mixed-lineage leukemia (MLL)* occur in 5–10% of adult acute leukemias and 70% of therapy-related AML, particularly following treatment with topoisomerase II inhibitors, and is associated with a poor prognosis [54, 55]. Menin is a scaffolding protein that functions as an essential cofactor of transcription factors such as NPM1 and chromatin regulators such as KMT2A [54]. Menin inhibitors block the binding of menin to KMT2A fusion proteins in KMT2A rearranged leukemias to induce differentiation and apoptosis [56]. Menin inhibitors are also active in *NPM1*-mutated AML, where they reverse aberrant gene expression mediated by *HOX* genes and MEIS1 [57, 58]. A phase 1 trial with the menin inhibitor SNDX-5613 and MI-3454 is currently underway.

APR-246 In AML, inactivating mutations in the *TP53* gene occur in 7–18% of patients with newly diagnosed AML and are associated with poor outcomes, particularly in patients with other poor prognostic features including complex karyotype and therapy-related disease [59–61]. APR-246 is a prodrug that is converted to the Michael acceptor methylene quinuclidinone, which covalently binds cysteine residues on mutated p53, leading to refolding and restoration of p53 function [62, 63]. In a phase 2 study of APR-246 in combination with azacitidine in patients with TP53-mutant MDS and AML, 75% responded and 56% achieved a CR with seven out of nine patients achieving a complete cytogenetic CR and clearance of TP53 mutations [64]. A phase 3 trial with the combination is currently ongoing.

4.7 Antibody-Based Therapies and Immunotherapies

4.7.1 Antibody-Based Therapy

BiTEs (Bispecific T-cell engagers) simultaneously bind antigens on leukemic cells and CD3 + T cells, allowing for recognition and elimination by cytotoxic T lymphocytes. The development of BiTEs in AML has been spurred by the success of the CD19/CD3 BiTE blinatumomab, which is approved for R/R ALL and ALL with minimal residual disease [65, 66].

AMG 330 (CD33/CD3 BiTE) and AMG 427 (FLT3/CD3 BiTE) are bispecific T cell engager that bind CD33 or FLT3 on myeloid blasts and CD3 on T cells. Preliminary results from a phase 1 study of unselected patients with R/R AML showed promising response rates after treatment with AMG 330 of 19%. Similar to other BiTEs, a reversible cytokine release syndrome was a common adverse event, occurring in 67% of patients treated in the phase 1 study [67]. **IMGN 632** is an antibody–drug conjugate consisting of a CD123 antibody linked to a DNA-alkylating indolino-benzodiazepine dimer (IGN) via a protease cleavable linker [68]. CD123 is highly expressed on leukemic stem cells capable of initiating and maintaining AML [69, 70]. In a phase 1 study of patients with CD123 + R/R AML, IMGN 632 led to responses in 20% of patients, and responses were enriched among patients with adverse risk disease (62% of responding patients) and primary induction failure (23% of responding patients). Dose-limiting toxicities included reversible veno-occlusive disease ($n = 2$) and prolonged neutropenia ($n = 1$) [71]. A phase 1b/2 study evaluating IMGN alone and in combination with venetoclax in CD123 + AML is currently underway [72].

Flotetuzumab is a bispecific dual-affinity re-targeting (DART) antibody-based molecule that binds CD3 on T-cells and CD123 on leukemic stem cells. Treatment with flotetuzumab in a phase 1 stuty of R/R AML led to an ORR of 24% and a CR/CRh rate of 18% but demonstrated higher responses among patients with primary induction failure and early relapse (ORR 30% and CR/CRh 27%) [73]. Biomarker analysis demonstrated that achievement of complete response correlated with higher levels of immune infiltration and expression of immune-related genes. Both CD123 expression and immune infiltration were higher in patients with primary induction failure and early relapse when compared to late relapsing patients [73].

Cusatuzumab is a monoclonal antibody targeting CD70 that induces antibody-dependent cell-mediated cytotoxicity to eradicate leukemic stem cells. Upregulation of CD70 after treatment with hypomethylating agents and subsequent cell-autonomous CD70/CD27 signaling triggers symmetric cell division and

Table 4.1 2017 ELN risk stratification by genetics

Risk category*	Genetic abnormality
Favorable	t(8;21)(q22;q22.1); *RUNX1-RUNX1T1* inv(16)(p13.1q22) or t(16;16)(p13.1;q22); *CBFB-MYH11* Mutated *NPM1* without *FLT3*-ITD or with *FLT3*-ITD^{low}† Biallelic mutated *CEBPA*
Intermediate	Mutated *NPM1* and *FLT3*-ITD^{high}† Wild-type *NPM1* without *FLT3*-ITD or with *FLT3*-ITD^{low}† (without adverse-risk genetic lesions) t(9;11) (p21.3;q23.3); *MLLT3-KMT2A*‡Cytogenetic abnormalities not classified as favorable or adverse

Adverse	t(6;9)(p23;q34.1); *DEK-NUP214*t(v;11q23.3); *KMT2A* rearranged
	t(9;22)(q34.1;q11.2); *BCR-ABL1*
	inv(3)(q21.3q26.2) or t(3;3)(q21.3;q26.2); *GATA2,MECOM(EVI1)*–5 or del (5q); −7; −17/abn(17p)Complex karyotype,§ monosomal karyotype‖
	Wild-type *NPM1* and *FLT3-ITD*^{high}†
	Mutated *RUNX1*{
	Mutated *ASXL1*{
	Mutated *TP53*#

†Low, low allelic ratio (,0.5); high, high allelic ratio ($0.5) by semiquantitative assessment of FLT3-ITD allelic ratio

‡The presence of t(9;11)(p21.3;q23.3) takes precedence over rare, concurrent adverse-risk gene mutations

§Three or more unrelated chromosome abnormalities in the absence of 1 of the WHO-designated recurring translocations or inversions, that is, t(8;21), inv(16) or t(16;16), t(9;11), t(v;11)(v;q23.3), t(6;9), inv(3) or t(3;3); AML with BCR-ABL1

‖Defined by the presence of 1 single monosomy (excluding loss of X or Y) in association with at least 1 additional monosomy or structural chromosome abnormality (excluding core-binding factor AML)

{These markers should not be used as an adverse prognostic marker if they co-occur with favorable-risk AML subtypes

Adapted from Dohner et al. Blood 2017; 129: 424–47

proliferation of leukemic stem cells [74]. In a phase 1 study of previously untreated elderly patients with AML, Cusatuzumab in combination with azacytidine induced CR/CRi in ten out of twelve patients [75]. The phase 2 CULMINATE trial is currently underway.

Magrolimab (Hu5F9-G4) is a humanized IgG4 targeting CD47 in order to enable phagocytosis of MDS or AML cells. CD47 is a transmembrane protein that functions as an anti-phagocytic or "do not eat me" signal by binding the inhibitory receptor signal-regulatory protein alpha (SIRPα) on macrophages [76]. In a phase Ib study of patients with untreated very high-risk MDS or AML patients unfit for chemotherapy, the ORR was 64% and the CR rate was 40%. Among patients with *TP53*-mutated AML, the CR + CRi rate was 75 with 50% of responders achieving MRD negativity by flow cytometry [77].

4.8 Chimeric Antigen Receptor (CAR) Modified Cellular Therapy

Chimeric antigen receptors (CAR) are engineered extracellular receptors joined to intracellular signaling domains that reprogram immune cells for therapeutic purposes [78, 79]. Significant progress was made with second-generation CARs, which included CD28 or 41BB-costimulatory domains to enable effective immune responses [79]. CAR therapy targeting CD19 has demonstrated marked activity in B-cell malignancies, resulting in approval of tisagenlecleucel (Kymriah) for pediatric B-ALL that is refractory or in second or later relapse and axicabtagene ciloleucel (Yescarta) in large B-cell lymphomas after 2 or more lines of systemic therapy [80, 81]. In AML, the ideal CAR target that is highly expressed in myeloid blasts and spares normal myeloid progenitor cells and vital tissues has not yet been identified [82]. It appears that CD33 and CD123 are attractive CAR targets although these antigens are expressed in both malignant and healthy cells [83, 84]. Since CD123 is expressed on both leukemia-initiating cells as well as on the healthy stem and progenitor cells, marrow aplasia a possibility with such approaches that may necessitate alloSCT to restore hematopoiesis [85]. An alternative approach currently in clinical development is the use of genetically modified donor allografts that lack expression of CAR targets (e.g., CD33), followed by administration of anti-CD33 CARs after transplantation [86]. The persistence of CARs post-transplant enables immune surveillance and memory to promote sustained remission. Toxicities of current CAR therapies particularly cytokine release syndrome and neurotoxicity are challenges in AML where the majority of relapsed patients are older and have comorbidities (Table 4.1).

References

1. Burnett AK et al (2015) A randomized comparison of daunorubicin 90 mg/m^2 versus 60 mg/m^2 in AML induction: results from the UK NCRI AML17 trial in 1206 patients. Blood 125(25):3878–3885
2. Fernandez HF et al (2009) Anthracycline dose intensification in acute myeloid leukemia 361 (13):1249–1259
3. Othus M et al (2016) Prediction of CR following a second course of '7+3' in patients with newly diagnosed acute myeloid leukemia not in CR after a first course. Leukemia 30:1779
4. Kantarjian H (2016) Acute myeloid leukemia—major progress over four decades and glimpses into the future. Am J Hematol 91(1):131–145
5. Holowiecki J et al (2012) Cladribine, but not fludarabine, added to daunorubicin and cytarabine during induction prolongs survival of patients with acute myeloid leukemia: a multicenter, randomized phase III study. J Clin Oncol 30(20):2441–2448
6. Castaigne S et al (2012) Effect of gemtuzumab ozogamicin on survival of adult patients with de-novo acute myeloid leukaemia (ALFA-0701): a randomised, open-label, phase 3 study. Lancet 379(9825):1508–1516
7. Hills RK et al (2014) Addition of gemtuzumab ozogamicin to induction chemotherapy in adult patients with acute myeloid leukaemia: a meta-analysis of individual patient data from randomised controlled trials. Lancet Oncol 15(9):986–996
8. Stone RM et al (2017) Midostaurin plus chemotherapy for acute myeloid leukemia with a FLT3 mutation. N Engl J Med 377(5):454–464
9. Lancet JE et al (2018) CPX-351 (cytarabine and daunorubicin) Liposome for injection versus conventional cytarabine plus daunorubicin in older patients with newly diagnosed secondary acute myeloid leukemia. J Clin Oncol 36(26):2684–2692
10. Lancet JE et al (2016) Survival following allogeneic hematopoietic cell transplantation in older high-risk acute myeloid leukemia patients initially treated with CPX-351 liposome injection versus standard cytarabine and daunorubicin: subgroup analysis of a large phase III trial. Blood 128(22):906–906
11. Kantarjian HM et al (2012) Multicenter, randomized, open-label, phase III trial of decitabine versus patient choice, with physician advice, of either supportive care or low-dose cytarabine for the treatment of older patients with newly diagnosed acute myeloid leukemia. J Clin Oncol 30(21):2670–2677
12. Blum W et al (2010) Clinical response and miR-29b predictive significance in older AML patients treated with a 10-day schedule of decitabine. Proc Natl Acad Sci U S A 107 (16):7473–7478
13. Welch JS et al (2016) TP53 and decitabine in acute myeloid leukemia and myelodysplastic syndromes. N Engl J Med 375(21):2023–2036
14. Amadori S et al (2016) Gemtuzumab ozogamicin versus best supportive care in older patients with newly diagnosed acute myeloid leukemia unsuitable for intensive chemotherapy: results of the randomized phase III EORTC-GIMEMA AML-19 trial. J Clin Oncol 34(9):972–979
15. Cortes JE et al (2019) Randomized comparison of low dose cytarabine with or without glasdegib in patients with newly diagnosed acute myeloid leukemia or high-risk myelodysplastic syndrome. Leukemia 33(2):379–389
16. DiNardo CD et al (2018) Venetoclax combined with decitabine or azacitidine in treatment-naive, elderly patients with acute myeloid leukemia. Blood
17. DiNardo CD et al (2018) Safety and preliminary efficacy of venetoclax with decitabine or azacitidine in elderly patients with previously untreated acute myeloid leukaemia: a non-randomised, open-label, phase 1b study. Lancet Oncol 19(2):216–228
18. Wei AH et al (2019) Venetoclax combined with low-dose cytarabine for previously untreated patients with acute myeloid leukemia: results from a phase Ib/II study. J Clin Oncol 37 (15):1277–1284

19. Wei AH et al (2020) Venetoclax plus LDAC for newly diagnosed AML ineligible for intensive chemotherapy: a phase 3 randomized placebo-controlled trial. Blood 135(24):2137–2145

20. DiNardo CD et al (2020) Azacitidine and venetoclax in previously untreated acute myeloid leukemia 383(7):617–629

21. Döhner H et al (2017) Diagnosis and management of AML in adults: 2017 ELN recommendations from an international expert panel. Blood 129(4):424–447

22. Koreth J et al (2009) Allogeneic stem cell transplantation for acute myeloid leukemia in first complete remission: systematic review and meta-analysis of prospective clinical trials. JAMA 301(22):2349–2361

23. Mayer RJ et al (1994) Intensive postremission chemotherapy in adults with acute myeloid leukemia. Cancer and Leukemia Group B. N Engl J Med 331(14):896–903

24. Tallman MS et al (2000) Effect of postremission chemotherapy before human leukocyte antigen-identical sibling transplantation for acute myelogenous leukemia in first complete remission. Blood 96(4):1254–1258

25. Yeshurun M et al (2014) Impact of postremission consolidation chemotherapy on outcome after reduced-intensity conditioning allogeneic stem cell transplantation for patients with acute myeloid leukemia in first complete remission: a report from the Acute Leukemia Working Party of the European Group for Blood and Marrow Transplantation. Cancer 120 (6):855–863

26. Pasquini MC et al (2015) Results of a phase III randomized, multi-center study of allogeneic stem cell transplantation after high versus reduced intensity conditioning in patients with myelodysplastic syndrome (MDS) or acute myeloid leukemia (AML): blood and marrow transplant clinical trials network (BMT CTN) 0901. Blood 126(23):LBA-8-LBA-8

27. Jackson G et al (2001) A multicentre, open, non-comparative phase II study of a combination of fludarabine phosphate, cytarabine and granulocyte colony-stimulating factor in relapsed and refractory acute myeloid leukaemia and de novo refractory anaemia with excess of blasts in transformation. Br J Haematol 112(1):127–137

28. Amadori S et al (1991) Mitoxantrone, etoposide, and intermediate-dose cytarabine: an effective and tolerable regimen for the treatment of refractory acute myeloid leukemia. J Clin Oncol 9(7):1210–1214

29. Herzig RH et al (1985) High-dose cytosine arabinoside therapy with and without anthracycline antibiotics for remission reinduction of acute nonlymphoblastic leukemia. J Clin Oncol 3(7):992–997

30. Medeiros BC et al (2016) Isocitrate dehydrogenase mutations in myeloid malignancies. Leukemia 31:272

31. Stein EM et al (2017) Enasidenib in mutant *IDH2* relapsed or refractory acute myeloid leukemia. Blood 130(6):722–731

32. DiNardo CD et al (2018) Durable remissions with ivosidenib in IDH1-mutated relapsed or refractory AML. N Engl J Med 378(25):2386–2398

33. Stahl M et al (2018) Hypomethylating agents in relapsed and refractory AML: outcomes and their predictors in a large international patient cohort. Blood Adv 2(8):923–932

34. Levis M, Perl AE (2020) Gilteritinib: potent targeting of FLT3 mutations in AML. Blood Adv 4(6):1178–1191

35. Kottaridis PD et al (2001) The presence of a FLT3 internal tandem duplication in patients with acute myeloid leukemia (AML) adds important prognostic information to cytogenetic risk group and response to the first cycle of chemotherapy: analysis of 854 patients from the United Kingdom Medical Research Council AML 10 and 12 trials. Blood 98(6):1752–1759

36. Frohling S et al (2002) Prognostic significance of activating FLT3 mutations in younger adults (16–60 years) with acute myeloid leukemia and normal cytogenetics: a study of the AML Study Group Ulm. Blood 100(13):4372–4380

37. Tien F-M et al (2018) Hyperleukocytosis is associated with distinct genetic alterations and is an independent poor-risk factor in de novo acute myeloid leukemia patients 101(1):86–94

38. Kayser S et al (2009) Insertion of FLT3 internal tandem duplication in the tyrosine kinase domain-1 is associated with resistance to chemotherapy and inferior outcome. Blood 114 (12):2386–2392
39. Schlenk RF et al (2014) Differential impact of allelic ratio and insertion site in FLT3-ITD-positive AML with respect to allogeneic transplantation. Blood 124(23):3441–3449
40. Stirewalt DL et al (2006) Size of FLT3 internal tandem duplication has prognostic significance in patients with acute myeloid leukemia. Blood 107(9):3724–3726
41. Liu SB et al (2019) Impact of FLT3-ITD length on prognosis of acute myeloid leukemia. Haematologica 104(1):e9–e12
42. Knapper S et al (2017) A randomized assessment of adding the kinase inhibitor lestaurtinib to first-line chemotherapy for FLT3-mutated AML. Blood 129(9):1143–1154
43. Propper DJ et al (2001) Phase I and pharmacokinetic Study of PKC412, an inhibitor of protein kinase C. J Clin Oncol 19(5):1485–1492
44. O'Farrell AM et al (2003) An innovative phase I clinical study demonstrates inhibition of FLT3 phosphorylation by SU11248 in acute myeloid leukemia patients. Clin Cancer Res 9 (15):5465–5476
45. Schlenk RF et al (2019) Midostaurin added to chemotherapy and continued single-agent maintenance therapy in acute myeloid leukemia with FLT3-ITD. Blood 133(8):840–851
46. Liu Y, Gray NS (2006) Rational design of inhibitors that bind to inactive kinase conformations. Nat Chem Biol 2(7):358–364
47. Smith CC et al (2015) FLT3 D835 mutations confer differential resistance to type II FLT3 inhibitors. Leukemia 29(12):2390–2392
48. Smith CC et al (2017) Heterogeneous resistance to quizartinib in acute myeloid leukemia revealed by single-cell analysis. Blood 130(1):48–58
49. Cortes J, Perl AE, Dohner H et al (2018) Quizartinib, an FLT3 inhibitor, as monotherapy in patients with relapsed or refractory acute myeloid leukaemia: an open-label, multicentre, single-arm, phase 2 trial. Lancet Oncol 19(7):889–903
50. McMahon CM et al (2019) Clonal selection with RAS pathway activation mediates secondary clinical resistance to selective FLT3 inhibition in acute myeloid leukemia. Cancer Discov 9 (8):1050–1063
51. Zhang H et al (2019) Clinical resistance to crenolanib in acute myeloid leukemia due to diverse molecular mechanisms. Nat Commun 10(1):244
52. Bewersdorf JP et al (2020) Venetoclax as monotherapy and in combination with hypomethylating agents or low dose cytarabine in relapsed and treatment refractory acute myeloid leukemia: a systematic review and meta-analysis. Haematologica
53. DiNardo CD et al (2020) Molecular patterns of response and treatment failure after frontline venetoclax combinations in older patients with AML. Blood
54. Issa GC et al (2021) Therapeutic implications of menin inhibition in acute leukemias. Leukemia
55. Super HJ et al (1993) Rearrangements of the MLL gene in therapy-related acute myeloid leukemia in patients previously treated with agents targeting DNA-topoisomerase II. Blood 82 (12):3705–3711
56. Grembecka J et al (2012) Menin-MLL inhibitors reverse oncogenic activity of MLL fusion proteins in leukemia. Nat Chem Biol 8(3):277–284
57. Uckelmann HJ et al (2020) Therapeutic targeting of preleukemia cells in a mouse model of NPM1 mutant acute myeloid leukemia. Science 367(6477):586–590
58. Klossowski S et al (2020) Menin inhibitor MI-3454 induces remission in MLL1-rearranged and NPM1-mutated models of leukemia. J Clin Invest 130(2):981–997
59. Kadia TM et al (2016) TP53 mutations in newly diagnosed acute myeloid leukemia: clinicomolecular characteristics, response to therapy, and outcomes. Cancer 122(22):3484–3491

60. Hou HA et al (2015) TP53 mutations in de novo acute myeloid leukemia patients: longitudinal follow-ups show the mutation is stable during disease evolution. Blood Cancer J 5:e331
61. Rucker FG et al (2012) TP53 alterations in acute myeloid leukemia with complex karyotype correlate with specific copy number alterations, monosomal karyotype, and dismal outcome. Blood 119(9):2114–2121
62. Lambert JM et al (2009) PRIMA-1 reactivates mutant p53 by covalent binding to the core domain. Cancer Cell 15(5):376–388
63. Zhang Q et al (2018) APR-246 reactivates mutant p53 by targeting cysteines 124 and 277. Cell Death Dis 9(5):439
64. Cluzeau T et al (2019) APR-246 combined with azacitidine (AZA) in TP53 mutated myelodysplastic syndrome (MDS) and acute myeloid leukemia (AML). A phase 2 study by the Groupe Francophone Des Myélodysplasies (GFM). Blood 134(Supplement_1):677–677
65. Kantarjian H et al (2017) Blinatumomab versus chemotherapy for advanced acute lymphoblastic leukemia 376(9):836–847
66. Gokbuget N et al (2018) Blinatumomab for minimal residual disease in adults with B-cell precursor acute lymphoblastic leukemia. Blood 131(14):1522–1531
67. Ravandi F et al (2020) Updated results from phase I dose-escalation study of AMG 330, a bispecific T-cell engager molecule, in patients with relapsed/refractory acute myeloid leukemia (R/R AML). 38(15_suppl):7508–7508
68. Kovtun Y et al (2018) A CD123-targeting antibody-drug conjugate, IMGN632, designed to eradicate AML while sparing normal bone marrow cells. Blood Adv 2(8):848–858
69. Munoz L et al (2001) Interleukin-3 receptor alpha chain (CD123) is widely expressed in hematologic malignancies. Haematologica 86(12):1261–1269
70. Jordan CT et al (2000) The interleukin-3 receptor alpha chain is a unique marker for human acute myelogenous leukemia stem cells. Leukemia 14(10):1777–1784
71. Daver NG et al (2019) Clinical profile of IMGN632, a novel CD123-targeting antibody-drug conjugate (ADC), in patients with relapsed/refractory (R/R) acute myeloid leukemia (AML) or blastic plasmacytoid dendritic cell neoplasm (BPDCN). Blood 134(Supplement_1):734–734
72. Daver NG et al (2020) A phase Ib/II study of the CD123-targeting antibody-drug conjugate IMGN632 as monotherapy or in combination with venetoclax and/or azacitidine for patients with CD123-positive acute myeloid leukemia 38(15_suppl):TPS7564-TPS7564
73. Uy GL et al (2020) Flotetuzumab as salvage immunotherapy for refractory acute myeloid leukemia. Blood
74. Riether C et al (2017) CD70/CD27 signaling promotes blast stemness and is a viable therapeutic target in acute myeloid leukemia. J Exp Med 214(2):359–380
75. Ochsenbein AF et al (2019) Targeting CD70 with cusatuzumab eliminates acute myeloid leukemia stem cells in humans. Blood 134(Supplement_1):234–234
76. Chao MP et al (2019) Therapeutic targeting of the macrophage immune checkpoint CD47 in myeloid malignancies. Front Oncol 9:1380
77. Sallman DA et al (2020) Tolerability and efficacy of the first-in-class anti-CD47 antibody magrolimab combined with azacitidine in MDS and AML patients: Phase Ib results 38 (15_suppl):7507–7507
78. Ball B, Stein EM (2019) Which are the most promising targets for minimal residual disease-directed therapy in acute myeloid leukemia prior to allogeneic stem cell transplant? Haematologica 104(8):1521–1531
79. June CH, Sadelain M (2018) Chimeric antigen receptor therapy. N Engl J Med 379(1):64–73
80. Maude SL et al (2018) Tisagenlecleucel in children and young adults with b-cell lymphoblastic leukemia. N Engl J Med 378(5):439–448
81. Neelapu SS et al (2017) Axicabtagene ciloleucel CAR T-cell therapy in refractory large B-cell lymphoma 377(26):2531–2544

82. Perna F et al (2017) Integrating proteomics and transcriptomics for systematic combinatorial chimeric antigen receptor therapy of AML. Cancer Cell 32(4):506–519 e5
83. Ehninger A et al (2014) Distribution and levels of cell surface expression of CD33 and CD123 in acute myeloid leukemia. Blood Cancer J 4:e218
84. Testa U, Pelosi E, Frankel A (2014) CD 123 is a membrane biomarker and a therapeutic target in hematologic malignancies. Biomarker Res 2(4)
85. Gill S et al (2014) Preclinical targeting of human acute myeloid leukemia and myeloablation using chimeric antigen receptor-modified T cells. Blood 123(15):2343–2354
86. Kim MY et al (2018) Genetic inactivation of CD33 in hematopoietic stem cells to enable CAR T cell immunotherapy for acute myeloid leukemia. Cell 173(6):1439-1453.e19

Current Management and New Developments in the Treatment of ALL

5

Justin Darrah and Weili Sun

Contents

J. Darrah (✉)
Division of Hematology and Cellular Therapy, Cedars-Sinai Medical Center,
8700 Beverly Blvd, Los Angeles, CA 90048, USA
e-mail: justin.darrah@cshs.org

W. Sun
City of Hope National Medical Center, Duarte, CA, USA

© Springer Nature Switzerland AG 2021
V. Pullarkat and G. Marcucci (eds.), *Biology and Treatment of Leukemia and Bone
Marrow Neoplasms*, Cancer Treatment and Research 181,
https://doi.org/10.1007/978-3-030-78311-2_5

5.1 Case 1

5.1.1 Newly Diagnosed T-Cell Acute Lymphoblastic Leukemia (T-ALL)

A 29-year-old man presents to the emergency room with chest pain, cough, and fever. He was found to have a white blood cell count of 95,000/μl with 85% blasts. His uric acid was 9.1 mg/dL. A chest X-ray demonstrated a large anterior mediastinal mass. He was diagnosed with T-ALL by peripheral blood morphology and flow cytometry. Leukemia blasts had normal karyotype and a lumbar puncture showed CNS1—no identifiable leukemia cells. He developed tumor lysis syndrome shortly after initiation of induction chemotherapy that was successfully managed by hydration, diuretics, and rasburicase. An end of induction bone marrow evaluation demonstrated complete remission (CR), but minimal residual disease (MRD) was 0.5% by multi-color flow cytometry. He wanted to know if an allogeneic hematopoietic stem cell transplant (allo-HCT) was necessary.

5.1.2 Discussion

Clinical presentation and diagnostic workup. T-ALL is a very aggressive leukemia that generally presents with a large tumor burden including leukocytosis and a large mediastinal mass. Some patients can develop tumor lysis syndrome at presentation [1]. A large mediastinal mass can cause obstruction and compression of vital mediastinal structures, leading to respiratory and hemodynamic compromise [2]. Therefore, it is important to recognize the signs and symptoms for early intervention. The diagnosis of T-ALL is made by morphology, immunophenotyping, and cytogenetic analysis of leukemia blasts. The leukemic blasts typically express CD3, TdT, and variable levels of CD1a, CD2, CD5, and CD7 [3]. A distinct subtype of T-ALL, called early T-cell precursor ALL (ETP-ALL), accounts for 7.4% of adult T-ALL. It is characterized by a unique immunophenotype cCD3+, sCD3−, CD1a−, CD2+, CD5−(dim), and positive for one or more stem cell/myeloid markers [4]. ETP-ALL is associated with a higher level of post-induction MRD and induction failure rate, leading to the poor long-term outcome if patients have received suboptimal therapy [5–9]. Many chromosomal translocations and genetic alterations have been identified in T-ALL. However, unlike with B-cell acute lymphoblastic leukemia (B-ALL), the prognostic significance of such changes in the context of modern MRD-guided risk-stratified chemotherapy remains unclear [8]. Compared to patients with B-ALL, patients with T-ALL are more likely to have CNS involvement at diagnosis (4.4 vs. 9.6%) [1]. Lumbar puncture and intrathecal chemotherapy are usually performed prior to the initiation of systemic chemotherapy as part of the diagnostic workup.

Treatment approaches. Several retrospective studies have demonstrated favorable outcomes of adolescents and young adults (AYA) with ALL when treated with a "pediatric-inspired" regimen [10]. The favorable result is seen in both B- and T-ALL [11–13]. The results of a prospective US cooperative group trial CALBG 10403 were reported utilizing an intensive pediatric regimen to treat AYA patients (17–39 years) [14]. The patients enrolled on this trial had a median event-free survival (EFS) of 78.1 months, significantly longer than the historical control of 30 months. The 3-year EFS was 59% and the estimated 3-year overall survival (OS) was 73%. Seventy-one T-ALL patients were included in this study and there was no significant difference in EFS and OS between patients with B- vs T-ALL. Only 20 of 263 patients received allo-HCT in CR1, suggesting that the excellent outcome was largely the result of chemotherapy. The pediatric inspired regimen consists of a 2–3 year multi-agent chemotherapy plan, usually including induction, consolidation, interim maintenance, delayed intensification, and maintenance. The most significant predictor of outcome in pediatric patients is end-of-consolidation MRD and treatment allocation is based on the MRD response [15–17]. Allo-HCT is not routinely used in pediatric patients but is considered for patients with induction failure or end-of-consolidation MRD $\geq$ 0.1% [8]. This response-based therapy is successful in the majority of patients, including patients with ETP-ALL [5–9]. The approaches to CNS-directed therapy vary. However, increasing data supports optimizing systemic chemotherapy in combination with intrathecal therapy, and cranial radiation can be successfully avoided in most patients [7, 18].

5.1.3 Recent Clinical Observations in Pediatrics

(1) Dexamethasone versus prednisone during induction. Both dexamethasone and prednisone have been used in the induction regimens for ALL. Dexamethasone has greater potency and CNS penetration, which is appealing in T-ALL. However, higher rates of infection and increased risk of avascular necrosis have been observed in dexamethasone-based regimens [19]. Several recent studies supported the use of dexamethasone in T-ALL [20–22]. In the AEIOP-BFM-2000 trial, patients were randomized to receive dexamethasone or prednisone during induction [23]. In good response T-ALL patients, dexamethasone resulted in a reduction of relapse from 17 to 7%, a significant improvement of EFS (dexamethasone 87.8% vs. prednisone 79.2%), and OS (dexamethasone 91.4% vs. prednisone 82.6%). However, higher toxicity and treatment-related mortality were observed in older patients.

(2) Escalating methotrexate (MTX) with asparaginase was superior to high-dose (HD) MTX in T-ALL. HD-MTX (5 g/m^2/dose) has demonstrated improved outcomes in high-risk B-ALL in children [24]. To investigate the efficacy of HD-MTX in T-ALL, the Children's Oncology Group (COG) AALL0434 trial randomized T-ALL patients (1–31 years) to receive HD-MTX versus Capizzi-style escalating MTX with 2 doses of PEG-asparaginase during interim maintenance [16]. Patients receiving the escalating MTX regimen demonstrated improved 4-year EFS of 92.5

versus 86.1% in HD-MTX group. The improved EFS was due to the reduction of marrow and CNS relapse.

(3) Nelarabine improved disease-free survival (DFS) in T-ALL. Nelarabine is a pro-drug of Ara-G that has been approved by the FDA to treat relapsed/refractory T-ALL [25, 26]. To evaluate the efficacy in newly diagnosed patients, the intermediate and high-risk patients enrolled on COG AALL0434 were randomized to receive nelarabine during consolidation, delayed intensification, and maintenance [16]. Patients receiving nelarabine demonstrated a superior 4-year DFS (88.9 vs. 83.3%) compared to those randomized without nelarabine [27]. The overall toxicity was acceptable and not significantly different between both arms.

Unsolved questions in adult patients. In pediatric studies, higher toxicities were observed with increasing age. Adult patients demonstrated more toxicities related to asparaginase, an important component of pediatric regimens. CALGB 10403 (utilizing prednisone and escalating dose MTX) demonstrated a tolerable safety profile in patients <40 years of age with an overall 3% ($n = 8$) treatment-related mortality and only two post-remission deaths [14]. However, there is uncertainty regarding the upper age limit for adults using a "pediatric-inspired" regimen. Some studies have demonstrated safe adaptation of a "pediatric-inspired" regimen in adult patients up to age 50–60 years of age [28, 29]. How to safely incorporate the new pediatric study results to treat adult patients remains unclear.

5.2 Case 2

5.2.1 Philadelphia Chromosome-Negative (Ph-Negative) B-Cell Acute Lymphoblastic Leukemia (B-ALL)

A 26-year-old man with no prior medical history presents to his primary care physician with symptoms of weakness, fatigue, loss of appetite, and a 10-lb weight loss over approximately four weeks. Initial workup included a CBC which showed a platelet count of 57,000/uL, hemoglobin 7.8 g/dL and a white blood cell count of 97,000/uL with 48% blasts. Subsequent workup with a diagnostic bone marrow biopsy showed 80% cellularity with 90% blasts. The blasts were positive for CD10, CD19, CD20, CD22, CD34, CD79a, and HLA-DR. They were negative for cCD3 and myeloperoxidase. Cytogenetics showed 46,XY t(4;11). BCR-ABL translocation was not identified. He was diagnosed with Ph-negative precursor B-ALL.

5.2.2 Which Treatment Regimen Should Be Used?

There is no standard treatment regimen for Ph-negative B-ALL. Many regimens are adapted from pediatric regimens and use a combination of an anthracycline, a corticosteroid, and vincristine. Cyclophosphamide, cytarabine, and asparaginase

Table 5.1 Commonly used ALL treatment regimens. DFS = median disease-free survival, EFS = median event-free survival, OS = median overall survival, CR = complete remission

Regimen (year)	Patients	Age range (median)	DFS (follow-up)	EFS (follow-up)	OS (follow-up)	CR
CALGB 10403 (2019) [14]	295	17–39 (24)	48% (36 months)	59% (36 months)	73% (36 months)	89%
Dana Farber Cancer Institute (DFCI) (2015) [52]	92	18–50 (28)	69% (48 months)	58% (48 months)	67% (48 months)	85%
GRAALL-2003 (2009) [28]	225	15–60 (31)	59%	55% (42 months)	60% (42 months)	93.5%
GRAALL-2005 (2018) [53]	787	18–59 (36.1)	–	52.2% (60 months)	58.5% (60 months)	91.9%
PETHEMA ALL-96 (2008) [54]	81	15–30 (20)	–	61% (72 months)	69% (72 months)	98%
Hyper-CVAD (2000) [55]	204	16–79 (39.5)	–	–	39% (60 months)	91%
USC ALL (2014) [29]	51	18–57 (32)	58% (84 months)	–	51% (84 months)	96%
Linker (2002) [56]	84	16–59 (27)	54% (60 months)	48% (60 months)	47% (60 months)	93%
CALGB 8811 (1995) [57]	197	16–80 (32)	–	–	50% (36 months)	85%
MRC UKALLXII/ECOG 2993 (2005) [58]	1521	15–59 (–)	–	–	38% (60 months)	91%

may also be included. A summary of the most commonly used regimens is provided in Table 5.1. These regimens have not been directly compared in prospective clinical trials and thus it is not known if one regimen provides superior outcomes to others. When possible, a pediatric-inspired regimen should be used as they have collectively been shown to provide better outcomes than adult regimens. In one meta-analysis of 11 trials treating adolescents and young adults (AYA) patients aged 16–39 years, those treated with pediatric-inspired regimens had a significant reduction in all-cause mortality (RR 0.59, 95% CI 0.52–0.66) and relapse rate (RR 0.51, 95% CI 0.39–0.66, $I^2 = 54\%$) as well as significant improvements in CR rate (RR 1.05, 95% CI 1.01–1.10, $I^2 = 55\%$) and EFS (RR 1.66, 95% CI 1.39–1.99, $I^2 = 61\%$) when compared to patients treated with conventional adult regimens [102]. Given the high propensity for CNS involvement, early and frequent CNS prophylaxis should also be incorporated into treatment. As this patient belongs to the AYA age group and has no medical comorbidities, he should be treated with a pediatric-inspired induction regimen.

Philadelphia chromosome-like (Ph-like) ALL is a subtype of ALL that has a gene expression profile similar to Philadelphia chromosome-positive (Ph-positive)

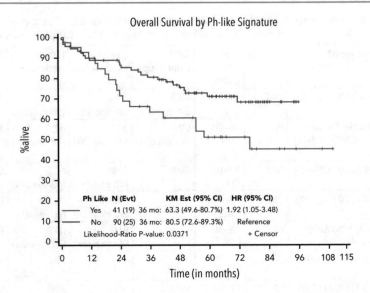

Fig. 5.1 Overall survival based on Ph-like signature [14]

ALL but lacks the BCR-ABL1 gene fusion that defines Ph-positive ALL (see Chap. 2 for the biology of Ph-like ALL). It occurs in approximately 20–30% of adult patients and is associated with poor outcomes [14, 103, 104]. In the CALGB 10403 study, estimated 3-year EFS was 42% (95% CI, 29–61%) for patients with Ph-like ALL compared to 69% (95% CI, 60–80%) for those with Ph-negative ALL (HR, 2.06; log-rank $P = 0.008$), and 3-year OS rate was 63% (95% CI, 50–81%) for patients with Ph-like ALL compared to 81% (95% CI, 73–89%) for those with Ph-negative ALL (Fig. 5.1) [14]. Ph-like ALL is typically treated with regimens similar to those used for Ph-negative ALL. Patients with Ph-like ALL tend to have a relatively high rate of MRD positivity at the end of induction chemotherapy, and those who achieve MRD negativity have a high risk of relapse [103, 104]. Therefore, consolidation with alloHCT should be considered in eligible patients with Ph-like ALL. Targeted therapy for ABL-class or JAK-STAT pathway mutations may be of benefit and is currently under investigation.

5.2.3 Should Asparaginase Be Included?

Asparaginase is a critical component of pediatric and pediatric-inspired treatment regimens. In AYA patients, the use of asparaginase has been associated with a significant improvement in DFS and overall survival [30]. However, asparaginase is less well tolerated in adults. Therefore, patients must be closely monitored during treatment. Typically, asparaginase is given up to the age of 40, however, some studies have successfully treated patients with asparaginase up to the age of

60 with appropriate dose modification, suggesting this may be possible when carefully administered in select patients [28, 29]. Patients should be monitored closely for asparaginase toxicity. Toxicities from asparaginase include bleeding, thrombosis, hepatotoxicity, hyperglycemia, pancreatitis, and hypersensitivity reactions [31, 32]. An asparaginase-containing treatment regimen should be used for the treatment of the patient in this case.

5.2.4 Should Rituximab Be Used?

In a single-center study of patients with Ph-negative precursor B-ALL, those under the age of 60 years had a significantly improved overall survival (75 vs. 47%; $P = 0.003$) and 3-year CR duration (70 vs. 38%; $P < 0.001$) when rituximab was added to the hyper-CVAD regimen (Fig. 5.2) [33]. The survival benefit was not observed in patients over the age of 60 years due to increased deaths after CR in the rituximab treated group, predominantly due to infectious causes [33]. In the GRAALL-R 2005 study, the addition of rituximab in patients aged 18–59 years with CD20-positive Ph-negative precursor B-ALL resulted in a lower incidence of relapse (18 vs. 32%; $p = 0.02$) and greater event-free survival (65% vs 52%; $p = 0.04$) at 2 years. There was no statistically significant improvement in overall survival among all patients, however a survival benefit was observed in the subset of patients undergoing allogeneic stem cell transplant in first remission (hazard ratio, 0.55; 95% CI, 0.34–0.91; $P = 0.02$). The incidence of severe adverse events did not differ between groups [34]. Based on these findings, rituximab should be included in the treatment of patients with Ph-negative precursor B-ALL, particularly those under the age of 60. Since this patient has CD20+ precursor B-ALL, he would benefit from the addition of rituximab.

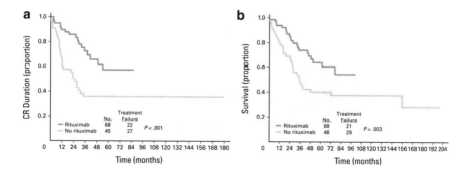

Fig. 5.2 Outcomes for patients younger than 60 years with Philadelphia-negative pre-B ALL. In the CD20-positive subset, **a** complete remission duration by therapy and **b** survival by therapy [33]

5.2.5 When Should Allogeneic Stem Cell Transplant Be Considered?

Patients at high risk of relapse after treatment should be considered for an allogeneic stem cell transplant. Among patients with Ph-negative ALL, MRD has emerged as the single most important risk factor for relapse. In the CALGB 10403 study, patients who were MRD-negative at the end of induction had a three-year DFS of 85% (95% CI, 74–98%) compared with 54% (95% CI, 41–71%; $P = 0.001$) for patients who were MRD-positive (Fig. 5.3) [14]. Similarly, in the combined analysis of the GMALL 06/99 and 07/03 studies, patients with persistent quantifiable MRD positivity ($\geq 10^{-4}$) after consolidation chemotherapy (week 16) had a significantly lower probability of obtaining a continuous CR at 5 years ($35\% \pm 5\%$ vs. $74\% \pm 3\%$; $P < 0.0001$). When patients undergoing stem cell transplant in first CR were excluded, this was even more pronounced (12 vs. 70%; $P < 0.0001$). Likewise, the overall survival was significantly lower in all patients with MRD positivity ($42\% \pm 5\%$ vs. $80\% \pm 3\%$; $P < 0.0001$) and when patients who underwent stem cell transplant in first CR were excluded ($33\% \pm 7\%$ vs. $81\% \pm 3\%$; $P < 0.0001$) (Figs. 5.4 and 5.5) [36]. In the GRAALL-2003/2005 trials, patients with ALL treated with the GRAAL protocol who were MRD-positive ($\geq 10^{-3}$) at the end of induction had a better relapse-free survival

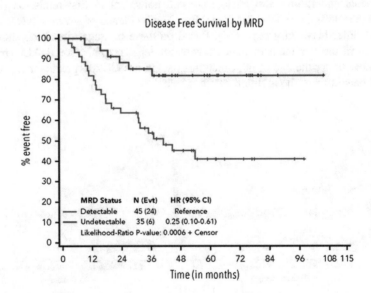

Fig. 5.3 Three-year DFS for patients with undetectable MRD compared to patients with detectable MRD at the end of induction [14]

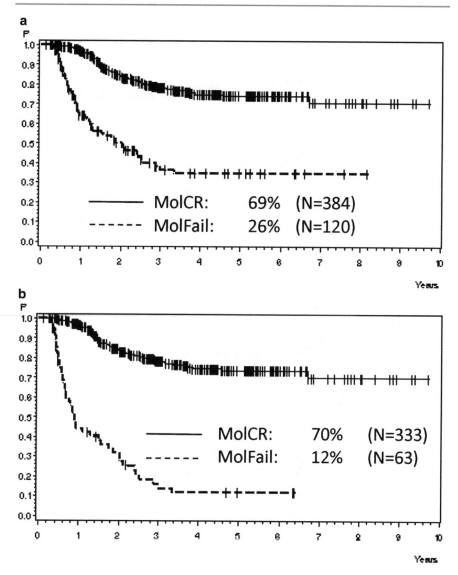

Fig. 5.4 Probability of continuous CR **a** in all patients and **b** with the exclusion of patients undergoing stem cell transplant in first CR [36]

(hazard ratio [HR] 0.40; 95% CI 0.23–0.69; $p = 0.001$) and overall survival (HR 0.41; 95% CI 0.23–0.74; $p = 0.002$) if they underwent allogeneic stem cell transplant in first CR [35], suggesting that allogeneic stem cell transplant improves outcomes in these high-risk patients. While the exact timing and MRD cutoff value to be used are still being elucidated, given the universally poor outcomes

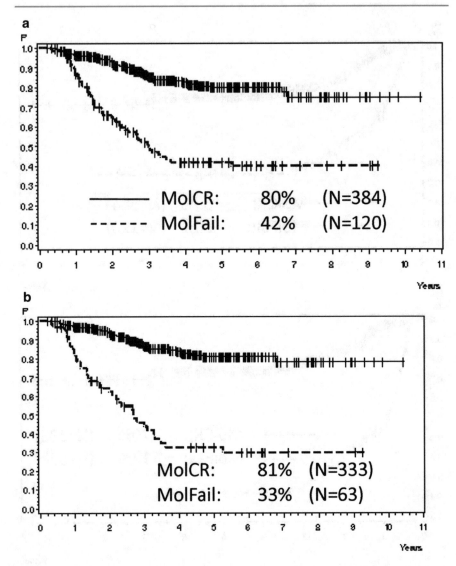

Fig. 5.5 Probability of survival **a** in all patients and **b** with the exclusion of patients undergoing stem cell transplant in first CR [36]

demonstrated in patients who have quantifiable MRD after induction and/or consolidation, these patients should be considered for allogeneic stem cell transplant in first CR when possible. Other clinical factors that have traditionally indicated high-risk disease include high white blood cell count at diagnosis (>30 × 10⁹/L in B-ALL or >100 × 10⁹/L in T-ALL), Ph-like gene expression profile, progenitor B-cell immunophenotype, *MLL* gene rearrangement (e.g., t(4;11)), *IKZF1* gene deletion, t(1;19) chromosomal translocation, low hypodiploidy/near triploidy, age >60 years, CNS involvement, and time to obtain CR > 4 weeks [37]. However, the GRAALL-2003/2005 trials identified the *IKZF1* gene deletion, *MLL* gene rearrangement, and MRD $\geq 10^{-4}$ at 6 weeks after induction start as the most significant factors for identifying high-risk patients with B-cell precursor ALL [39]. Because the patient, in this case, has the t(4;11) *MLL* gene rearrangement, he should undergo an allogeneic stem cell transplant in first CR if a suitable donor can be identified.

5.3 Case 3

5.3.1 Philadelphia Chromosome-Positive (Ph-Positive) B-Cell Acute Lymphoblastic Leukemia (B-ALL)

A 54-year-old woman with a history of hypertension and diabetes presents to the emergency room with symptoms of dyspnea on exertion and fatigue. Initial evaluation showed a platelet count of 88,000/μL, hemoglobin 4.1 g/dL, and a white cell count of 22,600/μL. A bone marrow biopsy was performed and showed a hypercellular bone marrow with 42% blasts. Flow cytometry showed expression of CD19, CD22, CD34, CD38, and HLA-DR. *BCR–ABL* P190 fusion was detected in 70.8% of the cells. She was diagnosed with Ph-positive B-ALL.

5.3.2 Which Induction Regimen Should Be Used?

Induction therapy for Ph-positive B-ALL should include a *BCR-ABL1* tyrosine kinase inhibitor (TKI) in addition to chemotherapy. The GRAAPH-2005 study compared imatinib plus a lower intensity induction chemotherapy regimen of weekly vincristine + dexamethasone versus imatinib plus Hyper-CVAD. All patients received imatinib, methotrexate, and cytarabine for the second cycle. After one cycle, the hematologic CR rate was higher in the vincristine + dexamethasone arm compared to the Hyper-CVAD arm (98.5 vs. 91.0%; $P = 0.006$). There were also less deaths in the vincristine + dexamethasone arm (60-day mortality 2.2 vs. 9%; $P = 0.017$). The major molecular response rate after two cycles demonstrated non-inferiority between the arms (66.1 vs. 64.5%; $P = 0.88$). There was no statistical difference between the arms in EFS, OS, or NRM [38]. Based on these findings of lower mortality and higher CR rate, with no difference in EFS, OS, and NRM, the lower intensity vincristine + dexamethasone regimen should be considered as the induction of choice in all patients who are eligible for TKI therapy. For older frail patients who are not suitable for induction chemotherapy, treatment with a TKI along with steroids alone could be considered. In this patient, treatment with the GRAAPH-2005 regimen would be reasonable.

5.3.3   Which TKI Should Be Used?

Imatinib, dasatinib, nilotinib, and ponatinib have all been demonstrated to be effective in the treatment of Ph-positive B-ALL. Imatinib was the first TKI evaluated for the treatment of Ph-positive B-ALL in combination with chemotherapy and demonstrated a CR rate of greater than 90% [40, 41]. However, imatinib does not adequately penetrate the blood–brain barrier, leaving the CNS vulnerable to leukemic infiltration. The second-generation TKIs dasatinib and nilotinib provide better CNS penetration [42]. In addition, they can also overcome many of the *BCR-ABL1* tyrosine kinase domain mutations that render imatinib ineffective, with the notable exception of the T315I mutation. Therefore, these second-generation TKIs have now become more commonly used in the front-line setting than imatinib.

When patients relapse after initial treatment, they often express the T315I kinase domain mutation [43–45]. Ponatinib, a third-generation TKI, is the only available TKI effective against the T315I mutation. Thus, ponatinib is frequently used in the relapsed setting. However, given the high rate of T315I mutation at the time of relapse and that some patients express the mutation at the time of diagnosis [46], there has been increasing interest in treating with ponatinib in the front-line setting. In one study evaluating the use of ponatinib in combination with Hyper-CVAD for frontline treatment, 100% of patients achieved a complete cytogenetic response, 95% achieved a major molecular response, and 78% had a complete molecular response. At a median of 3 weeks, 95% of patients were MRD-negative. At two years, EFS was 81% and OS was 80% [47]. The TKIs have never been directly compared in a randomized prospective trial, however, a meta-analysis of treatment with ponatinib plus chemotherapy versus earlier generation TKIs (imatinib, dasatinib, or nilotinib) plus chemotherapy suggested that ponatinib may produce better outcomes [48]. Regardless of which TKI is chosen, it is most effective when given continuously [49].

5.3.4   Post-Remission Treatment

While current treatment regimens for Ph-positive B-ALL result in a high CR rate, most patients will relapse if additional treatment is not given. The optimal post-remission therapy is not yet known and remains under investigation. The current standard remains allogeneic stem cell transplant in first CR for patients who are medically fit and have a suitable donor. Outcomes after allogeneic stem cell transplant have been shown to be superior to those after autologous stem cell transplant or chemotherapy alone [51], however, these data were established in the pre-TKI era. Newer data suggest that autologous stem cell transplant may be comparable to allogeneic stem cell transplant when TKI therapy is used, as discussed below, however this has not yet been validated in a prospective randomized study.

For patients who are unable to undergo allogeneic stem cell transplant, autologous stem cell transplant is a reasonable treatment option if used in conjunction with TKI therapy. Several studies have now demonstrated similar outcomes between allogeneic transplant versus autologous transplant followed by TKI maintenance, particularly if patients achieve a major molecular response (BCR-ABL1/ABL ratio of < 0.1% in the bone marrow) [38, 50]. However, it should be noted that these studies were not truly randomized trials. Rather, patients were offered autologous transplant if unable to undergo allogeneic transplant. In addition, TKI maintenance was given only to patients who underwent autologous stem cell transplant and not those who had an allogeneic transplant. Finally, TKI maintenance in these studies was with imatinib as opposed to the newer generation TKIs that are more commonly used today. It is unclear if outcomes would be different if TKI maintenance was used after allogeneic transplant as well, or if a more potent TKI was used. To that end, a trial is currently underway evaluating the use of dasatinib during induction followed by allogeneic stem cell transplant versus autologous stem cell transplant (CALGB 10701 Alliance). Nonetheless, until more data become available, autologous stem cell transplant is a reasonable secondary treatment option in patients unable to undergo allogeneic stem cell transplant.

Patients who are unsuitable for either allogeneic or autologous stem cell transplant should continue treatment with chemotherapy and TKI. The optimal TKI in this setting has not been determined, however a recent study combining Hyper-CVAD with ponatinib reported a 2 year EFS of 81% and 2 year OS of 80% [47]. Thus, this regimen would be a reasonable choice in the absence of medical contraindications to treatment.

Given her age and good overall health, this patient should be evaluated for allogeneic stem cell transplant. If a suitable donor cannot be identified, an autologous stem cell transplant followed by TKI maintenance could be considered.

5.4 Case 4

5.4.1 Relapsed ALL

A 24-year-old man was initially diagnosed with Ph-negative B-ALL at the age of 20 years and was treated with a pediatric chemotherapy regimen. He achieved MRD-negative remission at the end of induction. During maintenance therapy, he was found to have isolated bone marrow relapse. He achieved a second CR (CR2) after re-induction and received an allo-HCT from a matched unrelated donor. He developed a second bone marrow relapse 13 months post-HCT. He wants to know if there is any other treatment available.

5.4.2 Discussion

First relapse of ALL

Outcome in patients with first relapse of ALL. In first relapse of ALL, CR2 can be achieved in about 81–94% of pediatric patients [59–62], and a chemotherapy-alone approach can result in long-term survival in a subset of low-risk relapsed patients [59, 60, 63]. However, only approximately 40% of adult patients are able to achieve CR2, and this CR is generally transient if only receiving chemotherapy [64, 65]. Long-term DFS can be achieved in approximately 25% of patients with relapsed ALL, and in general occurs only with allo-HCT [64, 66]. Predictors for survival include duration of the first remission, response to reinduction therapy, ability to undergo HCT, disease burden at time of HCT, and age [64, 66–68].

Treatment approach in patients with first relapse of ALL. The initial approach to treat relapsed ALL in adults is to evaluate whether the patient is a potential candidate for allo-HCT. Referral to a transplant center and early donor identification is important since the duration of CR2 is generally short. The goal of salvage therapy is to achieve a CR2 (preferably MRD-negative) prior to HCT, since studies report improved outcomes if the patient has MRD-negative remission at the time of transplant [69].

Multiple salvage chemotherapy regimens have been used in adults with relapsed ALL, but none have been deemed as the standard of care. Common salvage chemotherapy regimens include high-dose cytarabine and fludarabine with G-CSF (FLAG), alone or in combination with an anthracycline; Hyper-CVAD with or without asparaginase; BFM based pediatric inspired regimen; Clofarabine based regimen; and liposomal vincristine [70–79]. In patients with T-ALL, treatment with nelarabine alone or in combination can be considered [25, 26].

If relapse occurs >12 months from initial diagnosis, retreating with the same previously successful induction regimen is reasonable. Otherwise, an alternative regimen may be considered. It is important to assess for CNS and testicular involvement at the time of systemic relapse and restart CNS prophylaxis with intrathecal chemotherapy. CNS relapse is often associated with a systemic relapse. Therefore, bone marrow biopsy and aspirate with MRD testing is necessary for disease evaluation. Even when there appears to be isolated CNS relapse, systemic treatment is recommended because the occurrence of a subsequent systemic relapse is likely [80–82]. In patients with CNS involvement, local radiation can be administered after systemic treatment. There has been no clear evidence suggesting the superiority of craniospinal radiation over cranial radiation, we recommend patients receive a dose of 18 Gy [82, 83].

New and emerging therapy in B-ALL. Most patients with relapsed/refractory ALL have chemotherapy-resistant disease. This has resulted in the development of treatments with alternative mechanisms of action. In 2017, the FDA approved three novel immunotherapies to treat patients with relapsed/refractory B-ALL which directly target surface antigens of leukemia blasts: inotuzumab ozogamicin, blinatumomab, and tisagenlecleucel.

Inotuzumab ozogamicin is an anti-CD22 monoclonal antibody conjugated to the cytotoxic antibiotic agent calicheamicin. After binding to CD22-positive leukemia blasts, the antibody complex is internalized and calicheamicin is released, inducing cell death [84]. In the phase III INO-VATE trial, adult patients with first relapsed B-ALL were randomized to receive inotuzumab ozogamicin or standard chemotherapy [84]. Compared to chemotherapy, the inotuzumab ozogamicin group demonstrated significantly higher response rates (CR + CRi 80.7 vs. 29.4%, $P < 0.001$; CR rate 35.8 vs. 17.4%), longer duration of remission (DOR, 4.6 months vs. 3.1 months, $p = 0.03$), longer progression-free survival (5 months vs. 1.8 months, $p = 0.04$), and longer OS (7.7 months vs. 6.7 months, $p = 0.04$). Hepatotoxicity, especially the rate of veno-occlusive disease (VOD), was markedly higher with the inotuzumab ozogamicin-treatment group, mostly occurring in patients who had undergone HCT before or after the therapy.

Blinatumomab is a bi-specific T-cell engager (BiTE) antibody that links CD19 + B-cells with CD3 + T-cells, leading to cytotoxic T-cell response against CD19 + leukemia blasts [85, 86]. In the phase III randomized TOWER trial, heavily pre-treated precursor B-ALL patients were randomly assigned to receive either blinatumomab or standard of care chemotherapy [87]. Similar to inotuzumab ozogamicin, blinatumomab showed significantly higher CR rates (34 vs. 16%, $p < 0.001$), longer DOR (7.3 months vs. 2.6 months), higher 6 months EFS (31 vs. 12%, $p < 0.0001$), and improved OS (7.7 months vs. 4 months, $p = 0.01$). The most common toxicities of blinatumomab included neurotoxicity and cytokine-release syndrome (CRS), similar to tisagenlecleucel, and will be discussed later in this chapter.

Multiply relapsed B-ALL

Outcome in patients with multiply relapsed ALL. The outcome for ALL patients with post-HCT relapse or multiple relapsed diseases is very poor. Approximately 50% of pediatric patients and 20% of adult patients can achieve CR following a second salvage chemotherapy attempt. However, the duration of remission is usually very short [65, 88]. There is no standard therapy available and we generally recommend enrollment in clinical trials for such patients. In the past several years, the promising results of ground-breaking chimeric antigen receptor (CAR) T-cell therapy have transformed how we treat these patients and we expect the outcome will improve in this extremely high-risk population [89]. Other novel therapies have also shown promise in this patient population. The combination of the BCL-2 inhibitor venetoclax and the BCL-2/BCL-X$_L$/BCL-W inhibitor navitoclax, with or without chemotherapy, was recently demonstrated to have significant efficacy. In a phase I trial of patients with relapsed/refractory ALL and lymphoblastic lymphoma, 18 of the 36 evaluated patients (50%) achieved a CR. Ten of the patients achieving CR were MRD-negative (55.6%) [105].

CD19 CAR T-cell therapy. CAR T-cell therapy is a novel adoptive cellular therapy that utilizes the patient's autologous T-cells, which are genetically engineered ex vivo to specifically recognize surface antigens expressed on tumor cells. The modified CAR T-cells are infused back into the patient, resulting in antigen recognition and rapid expansion of CAR T-cells, leading to leukemic cell killing [89]. CD19 is an antigen expressed in almost all B-cell ALL cells and has been widely used as a target in CAR T-cell therapy. Various CD19 CAR T-cell clinical trials in both children and adults have demonstrated similar high response rates and toxicities [90–96], although head-to-head comparisons across different trials is not possible due to the differences in manufacturing platforms and trial design [89]. CAR-T-cell therapy for ALL and its complications are discussed in further detail in Chap. 11.

Tisagenlecleucel is the first CD19 CAR T-cell therapy approved by the FDA to treat patients up to 25 years of age with B-cell ALL that is refractory or in second or later relapse. In the single-arm ELIANA trial, 75 pediatric and young adult patients with multiply relapsed/refractory ALL received tisagenlecleucel [96]. The CR rate within 3 months was 81%, all were MRD-negative CR. EFS was 73% at 6 months and 50% at 12 months. OS was 90% at 6 months and 76% at 12 months. These were extraordinary results when compared with historical data [65, 88]. Interestingly, only a small cohort of patients (<15%) underwent HCT after CAR T-cell therapy in the ELIANA trial indicating the possibility of long-term persistence of the CAR T-cells and durable remission without HCT consolidation. However, the persistence of the cells is unpredictable and the role of HCT after tisagenlecleucel is unclear. Therefore, until we have data to predict who will not relapse without subsequent therapy, patients who have not received prior HCT should be considered for consolidative HCT if they achieve remission after CAR T-cell therapy.

Both neurotoxicity and cytokine release syndrome (CRS), which can be potentially life-threatening, have been observed with tisagenlecleucel and blinatumomab. In the ELIANA trial, 40% of patients developed neurologic events, and 13% were severe ($\geq$ grade 3) including encephalopathy, confusion, and delirium. All CNS symptoms were transient. CRS was observed in 77% of patients, and 47% of patients were admitted to the ICU for the management of CRS. Severe CRS can be managed with tocilizumab, an anti-IL-6-receptor antibody that was simultaneously approved with tisagenlecleucel for the treatment of CAR T cell-associated CRS.

Other CAR T-cell therapies on the horizon. Although the outcome with tisagenlecleucel is impressive, some patients relapse with either CD19+ or CD19-disease, indicating different mechanisms of relapse [91, 97]. Alternative treatment options exploring different B-cell surface antigens (i.e., CD22, CD20, ROR1, and BAFF-R), or combination antigens (i.e., CD19/CD22, CD19/CD20) are ongoing [98–100]. In addition, some patients are unable to receive autologous CAR T-cells due to an inability to manufacture a usable product as a result of comorbidities or impaired T-cell function after prior chemotherapy. Those issues could potentially be avoided by the use of allogeneic or "off-the-shelf" CAR T-cells which are currently in development [101].

References

1. Marks DI, Paietta EM, Moorman AV et al (2009) T-cell acute lymphoblastic leukemia in adults: clinical features, immunophenotype, cytogenetics, and outcome from the large randomized prospective trial (UKALL XII/ECOG 2993). Blood 114(25):5136–5145
2. Lewis MA, Hendrickson AW, Moynihan TJ (2011) Oncologic emergencies: pathophysiology, presentation, diagnosis, and treatment. CA Cancer J Clin 61(5):287–314
3. Bene MC, Castoldi G, Knapp W et al (1995) Proposals for the immunological classification of acute leukemias. European Group for the Immunological Characterization of Leukemias (EGIL). Leukemia 9(10):1783–1786
4. Arber DA, Orazi A, Hasserjian R et al (2016) The 2016 revision to the World Health Organization classification of myeloid neoplasms and acute leukemia. Blood 127(20):2391–2405
5. Coustan-Smith E, Mullighan CG, Onciu M et al (2009) Early T-cell precursor leukaemia: a subtype of very high-risk acute lymphoblastic leukaemia. Lancet Oncol 10(2):147–156
6. Inukai T, Kiyokawa N, Campana D et al (2012) Clinical significance of early T-cell precursor acute lymphoblastic leukaemia: results of the Tokyo children's cancer study group study L99-15. Br J Haematol 156(3):358–365
7. Patrick K, Wade R, Goulden N et al (2014) Outcome for children and young people with Early T-cell precursor acute lymphoblastic leukaemia treated on a contemporary protocol, UKALL 2003. Br J Haematol 166(3):421–424
8. Raetz EA, Teachey DT (2016) T-cell acute lymphoblastic leukemia. Hematology Am Soc Hematol Educ Program 2016(1):580–588
9. Bond J, Graux C, Lhermitte L et al (2017) Early response-based therapy stratification improves survival in adult early thymic precursor acute lymphoblastic leukemia: a group for research on adult acute lymphoblastic leukemia study. J Clin Oncol 35(23):2683–2691
10. Boissel N, Sender LS (2015) Best practices in adolescent and young adult patients with acute lymphoblastic leukemia: a focus on asparaginase. J Adolesc Young Adult Oncol 4(3):118–128
11. Stock W, La M, Sanford B et al (2008) What determines the outcomes for adolescents and young adults with acute lymphoblastic leukemia treated on cooperative group protocols? A comparison of children's cancer group and cancer and leukemia group B studies. Blood 112 (5):1646–1654
12. Al-Khabori M, Minden MD, Yee KW et al (2010) Improved survival using an intensive, pediatric-based chemotherapy regimen in adults with T-cell acute lymphoblastic leukemia. Leuk Lymphoma 51(1):61–65
13. Ben Abdelali R, Asnafi V, Leguay T et al (2011) Pediatric-inspired intensified therapy of adult T-ALL reveals the favorable outcome of NOTCH1/FBXW7 mutations, but not of low ERG/BAALC expression: a GRAALL study. Blood 118(19):5099–5100
14. Stock W, Luger SM, Advani AS et al (2019) A pediatric regimen for older adolescents and young adults with acute lymphoblastic leukemia: results of CALGB 10403. Blood 133 (14):1548–1559
15. Schrappe M, Valsecchi MG, Bartram CR et al (2011) Late MRD response determines relapse risk overall and in subsets of childhood T-cell ALL: results of the AIEOP-BFM-ALL 2000 study. Blood 118(8):2077–2084
16. Winter SS, Dunsmore KP, Devidas M et al (2018) Improved survival for children and young adults with T-lineage acute lymphoblastic leukemia: results from the children's oncology group AALL0434 methotrexate randomization. J Clin Oncol 36(29):2926–2934
17. Pui CH, Pei D, Raimondi SC et al (2017) Clinical impact of minimal residual disease in children with different subtypes of acute lymphoblastic leukemia treated with response-adapted therapy. Leukemia 31(2):333–339
18. Pui CH, Campana D, Pei D et al (2009) Treating childhood acute lymphoblastic leukemia without cranial irradiation. N Engl J Med 360(26):2730–2741

19. Teuffel O, Kuster SP, Hunger SP et al (2011) Dexamethasone versus prednisone for induction therapy in childhood acute lymphoblastic leukemia: a systematic review and meta-analysis. Leukemia 25(8):1232–1238
20. Mitchell CD, Richards SM, Kinsey SE et al (2005) Benefit of dexamethasone compared with prednisolone for childhood acute lymphoblastic leukaemia: results of the UK Medical Research Council ALL97 randomized trial. Br J Haematol 129(6):734–745
21. Mitchell C, Richards S, Harrison CJ, Eden T (2010) Long-term follow-up of the United Kingdom medical research council protocols for childhood acute lymphoblastic leukaemia, 1980–2001. Leukemia 24(2):406–418
22. Vora A, Goulden N, Wade R et al (2013) Treatment reduction for children and young adults with low-risk acute lymphoblastic leukaemia defined by minimal residual disease (UKALL 2003): a randomised controlled trial. Lancet Oncol 14(3):199–209
23. Moricke A, Zimmermann M, Valsecchi MG et al (2016) Dexamethasone vs prednisone in induction treatment of pediatric ALL: results of the randomized trial AIEOP-BFM ALL 2000. Blood 127(17):2101–2112
24. Larsen EC, Devidas M, Chen S et al (2016) Dexamethasone and high-dose methotrexate improve outcome for children and young adults with high-risk B-acute lymphoblastic leukemia: a report from children's oncology group study AALL0232. J Clin Oncol 34 (20):2380–2388
25. DeAngelo DJ, Yu D, Johnson JL et al (2007) Nelarabine induces complete remissions in adults with relapsed or refractory T-lineage acute lymphoblastic leukemia or lymphoblastic lymphoma: cancer and leukemia group B study 19801. Blood 109(12):5136–5142
26. Gokbuget N, Basara N, Baurmann H et al (2011) High single-drug activity of nelarabine in relapsed T-lymphoblastic leukemia/lymphoma offers curative option with subsequent stem cell transplantation. Blood 118(13):3504–3511
27. Dunsmore KP, Winter S, Devidas M et al (2018) COG AALL0434: a randomized trial testing nelarabine in newly diagnosed t-cell malignancy. J Clin Oncol 36(15_suppl):10500–10500
28. Huguet F, Leguay T, Raffoux E et al (2009) Pediatric-inspired therapy in adults with Philadelphia chromosome-negative acute lymphoblastic leukemia: the GRAALL-2003 study. J Clin Oncol 27(6):911–918
29. Douer D, Aldoss I, Lunning MA et al (2014) Pharmacokinetics-based integration of multiple doses of intravenous pegaspargase in a pediatric regimen for adults with newly diagnosed acute lymphoblastic leukemia. J Clin Oncol 32(9):905–911
30. Wetzler M, Sanford BL, Kurtzberg J, Deoliveira D, Frankel SR, Powell BL, Kolitz JE, Bloomfield CD, Larson RA (2007) Effective asparagine depletion with pegylated asparaginase results in improved outcomes in adult acute lymphoblastic leukemia: cancer and leukemia group B Study 9511. Blood 109:4164–4167
31. Earl M (2009) Incidence and management of asparaginase-associated adverse events in patients with acute lymphoblastic leukemia. Clin Adv Hematol Oncol 7(9):600
32. Stock W, Douer D, Deangelo DJ et al (2011) Prevention and management of asparaginase/pegasparaginase-associated toxicities in adults and older adolescents: recommendations of an expert panel. Leuk Lymphoma 52:2237–2253
33. Thomas DA, O'brien S, Faderl S et al (2010) Chemoimmunotherapy with a modified hyper-CVAD and rituximab regimen improves outcome in de novo Philadelphia chromosome–negative precursor B-lineage acute lymphoblastic leukemia. J Clin Oncol 28:3880–3889
34. Maury S, Chevret S, Thomas X et al (2016) Rituximab in B-lineage adult acute lymphoblastic leukemia. N Engl J Med 375:1044–1053
35. Dhedin N, Huynh A, Maury S et al (2015) Role of allogeneic stem cell transplantation in adult patients with Ph-negative acute lymphoblastic leukemia. Blood 125:2486–2496

36. Gokbuget N, Kneba M, Raff T et al (2012) Adult patients with acute lymphoblastic leukemia and molecular failure display a poor prognosis and are candidates for stem cell transplantation and targeted therapies. Blood 120:1868–1876
37. Hoelzer D, Bassan R, Dombret H, Fielding A, Ribera JM, Buske C (2016) Acute lymphoblastic leukaemia in adult patients: ESMO Clinical Practice Guidelines for diagnosis, treatment and follow-up. Ann Oncol. https://doi.org/10.1093/annonc/mdw025
38. Chalandon Y, Thomas X, Hayette S et al (2015) Group for Research on Adult Acute Lymphoblastic Leukemia (GRAALL). Randomized study of reduced-intensity chemotherapy combined with imatinib in adults with Ph-positive acute lymphoblastic leukemia. Blood 125(24):3711–3719; Blood 126:1261–1261
39. Beldjord K, Chevret S, Asnafi V et al (2014) Oncogenetics and minimal residual disease are independent outcome predictors in adult patients with acute lymphoblastic leukemia. Blood 123:3739–3749
40. Thomas DA (2004) Treatment of Philadelphia chromosome-positive acute lymphocytic leukemia with hyper-CVAD and imatinib mesylate. Blood 103:4396–4407
41. Yanada M, Takeuchi J, Sugiura I et al (2006) High complete remission rate and promising outcome by combination of imatinib and chemotherapy for newly diagnosed BCR-ABL–positive acute lymphoblastic leukemia: a phase II study by the Japan adult leukemia study group. J Clin Oncol 24:460–466
42. Reinwald M, Schleyer E, Kiewe P et al (2014) Efficacy and pharmacologic data of second-generation tyrosine kinase inhibitor nilotinib in BCR-ABL-positive leukemia patients with central nervous system relapse after allogeneic stem cell transplantation. Biomed Res Int 2014:1–7
43. Foa R, Vitale A, Vignetti M et al (2011) Dasatinib as first-line treatment for adult patients with Philadelphia chromosome-positive acute lymphoblastic leukemia. Blood 118:6521–6528
44. Ravandi F, O'brien SM, Cortes JE et al (2015) Long-term follow-up of a phase 2 study of chemotherapy plus dasatinib for the initial treatment of patients with Philadelphia chromosome-positive acute lymphoblastic leukemia. Cancer 121:4158–4164
45. Soverini S, Benedittis CD, Papayannidis C et al (2013) Drug resistance and BCR-ABL kinase domain mutations in Philadelphia chromosome-positive acute lymphoblastic leukemia from the imatinib to the second-generation tyrosine kinase inhibitor era: The main changes are in the type of mutations, but not in the fr. Cancer 120:1002–1009
46. Soverini S, Vitale A, Poerio A et al (2010) Philadelphia-positive acute lymphoblastic leukemia patients already harbor BCR-ABL kinase domain mutations at low levels at the time of diagnosis. Haematologica 96:552–557
47. Jabbour E, Kantarjian H, Ravandi F et al (2015) Combination of hyper-CVAD with ponatinib as first-line therapy for patients with Philadelphia chromosome-positive acute lymphoblastic leukaemia: a single-centre, phase 2 study. Lancet Oncol 16:1547–1555
48. Jabbour E, Dersarkissian M, Duh MS et al (2018) Efficacy of ponatinib versus earlier generation tyrosine kinase inhibitors for front-line treatment of newly diagnosed Philadelphia-positive acute lymphoblastic leukemia. Clin Lymphoma Myeloma Leuk 18:257–265
49. Wassmann B (2006) Alternating versus concurrent schedules of imatinib and chemotherapy as front-line therapy for Philadelphia-positive acute lymphoblastic leukemia (Ph ALL). Blood 108:1469–1477
50. Wetzler M, Watson D, Stock W et al (2013) Autologous transplantation for Philadelphia chromosome-positive acute lymphoblastic leukemia achieves outcomes similar to allogeneic transplantation: results of CALGB Study 10001 (Alliance). Haematologica 99:111–115
51. Wrzesień-Kuś A, Robak T, Pluta A et al (2006) Outcome of treatment in adults with Philadelphia chromosome-positive and/or BCR–ABL-positive acute lymphoblastic leukemia —retrospective analysis of polish adult leukemia group (PALG). Ann Hematol 85:366–373

52. Deangelo DJ, Stevenson KE, Dahlberg SE et al (2014) Long-term outcome of a pediatric-inspired regimen used for adults aged 18–50 years with newly diagnosed acute lymphoblastic leukemia. Leukemia 29:526–534

53. Huguet F, Chevret S, Leguay T et al (2018) Intensified therapy of acute lymphoblastic leukemia in adults: report of the randomized GRAALL-2005 clinical trial. J Clin Oncol 36:2514–2523

54. Ribera J-M, Oriol A, Sanz M-A et al (2008) Comparison of the results of the treatment of adolescents and young adults with standard-risk acute lymphoblastic leukemia with the programa español de tratamiento en hematología pediatric-based protocol ALL-96. J Clin Oncol 26:1843–1849

55. Kantarjian HM, O'Brien S, Smith TL et al (2000) Results of treatment with hyper-CVAD, a dose-intensive regimen, in adult acute lymphocytic leukemia. J Clin Oncol 18:547–561

56. Linker C, Damon L, Ries C, Navarro W (2002) Intensified and shortened cyclical chemotherapy for adult acute lymphoblastic leukemia. J Clin Oncol 20:2464–2471

57. Larson RA, Dodge RK, Burns CP et al (1995) A five-drug remission induction regimen with intensive consolidation for adults with acute lymphoblastic leukemia: cancer and leukemia group B study 8811. Blood 85:2025–2037

58. Rowe JM (2005) Induction therapy for adults with acute lymphoblastic leukemia: results of more than 1500 patients from the international ALL trial: MRC UKALL XII/ECOG E2993. Blood 106:3760–3767

59. Tallen G, Ratei R, Mann G et al (2010) Long-term outcome in children with relapsed acute lymphoblastic leukemia after time-point and site-of-relapse stratification and intensified short-course multidrug chemotherapy: results of trial ALL-REZ BFM 90. J Clin Oncol 28 (14):2339–2347

60. Parker C, Waters R, Leighton C et al (2010) Effect of mitoxantrone on outcome of children with first relapse of acute lymphoblastic leukaemia (ALL R3): an open-label randomised trial. Lancet 376(9757):2009–2017

61. Raetz EA, Borowitz MJ, Devidas M et al (2008) Reinduction platform for children with first marrow relapse of acute lymphoblastic Leukemia: A children's oncology group study [corrected]. J Clin Oncol 26(24):3971–3978

62. Ko RH, Ji L, Barnette P et al (2010) Outcome of patients treated for relapsed or refractory acute lymphoblastic leukemia: a therapeutic advances in childhood leukemia consortium study. J Clin Oncol 28(4):648–654

63. Eapen M, Raetz E, Zhang MJ et al (2006) Outcomes after HLA-matched sibling transplantation or chemotherapy in children with B-precursor acute lymphoblastic leukemia in a second remission: a collaborative study of the children's oncology group and the center for international blood and marrow transplant research. Blood 107(12):4961–4967

64. Gokbuget N, Stanze D, Beck J et al (2012) Outcome of relapsed adult lymphoblastic leukemia depends on response to salvage chemotherapy, prognostic factors, and performance of stem cell transplantation. Blood 120(10):2032–2041

65. Gokbuget N, Dombret H, Ribera JM et al (2016) International reference analysis of outcomes in adults with B-precursor Ph-negative relapsed/refractory acute lymphoblastic leukemia. Haematologica 101(12):1524–1533

66. Fielding AK, Richards SM, Chopra R et al (2007) Outcome of 609 adults after relapse of acute lymphoblastic leukemia (ALL); an MRC UKALL12/ECOG 2993 study. Blood 109 (3):944–950

67. Oriol A, Vives S, Hernandez-Rivas JM et al (2010) Outcome after relapse of acute lymphoblastic leukemia in adult patients included in four consecutive risk-adapted trials by the PETHEMA Study Group. Haematologica 95(4):589–596

68. Duval M, Klein JP, He W et al (2010) Hematopoietic stem-cell transplantation for acute leukemia in relapse or primary induction failure. J Clin Oncol 28(23):3730–3738

69. Buckley SA, Appelbaum FR, Walter RB (2013) Prognostic and therapeutic implications of minimal residual disease at the time of transplantation in acute leukemia. Bone Marrow Transplant 48(5):630–641
70. Montillo M, Tedeschi A, Centurioni R, Leoni P (1997) Treatment of relapsed adult acute lymphoblastic leukemia with fludarabine and cytosine arabinoside followed by granulocyte colony-stimulating factor (FLAG-GCSF). Leuk Lymphoma 25(5–6):579–583
71. Specchia G, Pastore D, Carluccio P et al (2005) FLAG-IDA in the treatment of refractory/relapsed adult acute lymphoblastic leukemia. Ann Hematol 84(12):792–795
72. Faderl S, Thomas DA, O'Brien S et al (2011) Augmented hyper-CVAD based on dose-intensified vincristine, dexamethasone, and asparaginase in adult acute lymphoblastic leukemia salvage therapy. Clin Lymphoma Myeloma Leuk 11(1):54–59
73. Koller CA, Kantarjian HM, Thomas D et al (1997) The hyper-CVAD regimen improves outcome in relapsed acute lymphoblastic leukemia. Leukemia 11(12):2039–2044
74. Aldoss I, Pullarkat V, Patel R et al (2013) An effective reinduction regimen for first relapse of adult acute lymphoblastic leukemia. Med Oncol 30(4):744
75. Kantarjian H, Gandhi V, Cortes J et al (2003) Phase 2 clinical and pharmacologic study of clofarabine in patients with refractory or relapsed acute leukemia. Blood 102(7):2379–2386
76. Abbi KK, Rybka W, Ehmann WC, Claxton DF (2015) Phase I/II study of clofarabine, etoposide, and mitoxantrone in patients with refractory or relapsed acute leukemia. Clin Lymphoma Myeloma Leuk 15(1):41–46
77. Advani AS, Gundacker HM, Sala-Torra O et al (2010) Southwest oncology group study S0530: a phase 2 trial of clofarabine and cytarabine for relapsed or refractory acute lymphocytic leukaemia. Br J Haematol 151(5):430–434
78. Barba P, Sampol A, Calbacho M et al (2012) Clofarabine-based chemotherapy for relapsed/refractory adult acute lymphoblastic leukemia and lymphoblastic lymphoma. The Spanish experience. Am J Hematol 87(6):631–634
79. O'Brien S, Schiller G, Lister J et al (2013) High-dose vincristine sulfate liposome injection for advanced, relapsed, and refractory adult Philadelphia chromosome-negative acute lymphoblastic leukemia. J Clin Oncol 31(6):676–683
80. Gokbuget N, Hoelzer D (1998) Meningeosis leukaemica in adult acute lymphoblastic leukaemia. J Neurooncol 38(2–3):167–180
81. Ribeiro RC, Rivera GK, Hudson M et al (1995) An intensive re-treatment protocol for children with an isolated CNS relapse of acute lymphoblastic leukemia. J Clin Oncol 13(2):333–338
82. Ritchey AK, Pollock BH, Lauer SJ, Andejeski Y, Barredo J, Buchanan GR (1999) Improved survival of children with isolated CNS relapse of acute lymphoblastic leukemia: a pediatric oncology group study. J Clin Oncol 17(12):3745–3752
83. Barredo JC, Devidas M, Lauer SJ et al (2006) Isolated CNS relapse of acute lymphoblastic leukemia treated with intensive systemic chemotherapy and delayed CNS radiation: a pediatric oncology group study. J Clin Oncol 24(19):3142–3149
84. Kantarjian HM, DeAngelo DJ, Stelljes M et al (2016) Inotuzumab ozogamicin versus standard therapy for acute lymphoblastic leukemia. N Engl J Med 375(8):740–753
85. Topp MS, Gokbuget N, Zugmaier G et al (2014) Phase II trial of the anti-CD19 bispecific T cell-engager blinatumomab shows hematologic and molecular remissions in patients with relapsed or refractory B-precursor acute lymphoblastic leukemia. J Clin Oncol 32(36):4134–4140
86. Topp MS, Gokbuget N, Stein AS et al (2015) Safety and activity of blinatumomab for adult patients with relapsed or refractory B-precursor acute lymphoblastic leukaemia: a multicentre, single-arm, phase 2 study. Lancet Oncol 16(1):57–66
87. Kantarjian H, Stein A, Gokbuget N et al (2017) Blinatumomab versus chemotherapy for advanced acute lymphoblastic leukemia. N Engl J Med 376(9):836–847

88. Sun W, Malvar J, Sposto R et al (2018) Outcome of children with multiply relapsed B-cell acute lymphoblastic leukemia: a therapeutic advances in childhood leukemia & lymphoma study. Leukemia 32(11):2316–2325
89. Pehlivan KC, Duncan BB, Lee DW (2018) CAR-T cell therapy for acute lymphoblastic leukemia: transforming the treatment of relapsed and refractory disease. Curr Hematol Malig Rep 13(5):396–406
90. Davila ML, Riviere I, Wang X et al (2014) Efficacy and toxicity management of 19–28z CAR T cell therapy in B cell acute lymphoblastic leukemia. Sci Transl Med 6 (224):224ra225
91. Maude SL, Frey N, Shaw PA et al (2014) Chimeric antigen receptor T cells for sustained remissions in leukemia. N Engl J Med 371(16):1507–1517
92. Lee DW, Kochenderfer JN, Stetler-Stevenson M et al (2015) T cells expressing CD19 chimeric antigen receptors for acute lymphoblastic leukaemia in children and young adults: a phase 1 dose-escalation trial. Lancet 385(9967):517–528
93. Turtle CJ, Hanafi LA, Berger C et al (2016) CD19 CAR-T cells of defined CD4+:CD8+ composition in adult B cell ALL patients. J Clin Invest 126(6):2123–2138
94. Gardner RA, Finney O, Annesley C et al (2017) Intent-to-treat leukemia remission by CD19 CAR T cells of defined formulation and dose in children and young adults. Blood 129 (25):3322–3331
95. Park JH, Riviere I, Gonen M et al (2018) Long-term follow-up of CD19 CAR therapy in acute lymphoblastic leukemia. N Engl J Med 378(5):449–459
96. Maude SL, Laetsch TW, Buechner J et al (2018) Tisagenlecleucel in children and young adults with B-cell lymphoblastic leukemia. N Engl J Med 378(5):439–448
97. Sotillo E, Barrett DM, Black KL et al (2015) Convergence of acquired mutations and alternative splicing of CD19 enables resistance to CART-19 immunotherapy. Cancer Discov 5(12):1282–1295
98. Wang Y, Zhang WY, Han QW et al (2014) Effective response and delayed toxicities of refractory advanced diffuse large B-cell lymphoma treated by CD20-directed chimeric antigen receptor-modified T cells. Clin Immunol 155(2):160–175
99. Deniger DC, Yu J, Huls MH et al (2015) Sleeping beauty transposition of chimeric antigen receptors targeting receptor tyrosine kinase-like orphan receptor-1 (ROR1) into diverse memory T-cell populations. PLoS One 10(6):e0128151
100. Fry TJ, Shah NN, Orentas RJ et al (2018) CD22-targeted CAR T cells induce remission in B-ALL that is naive or resistant to CD19-targeted CAR immunotherapy. Nat Med 24(1):20–28
101. Qasim W, Zhan H, Samarasinghe S et al (2017) Molecular remission of infant B-ALL after infusion of universal TALEN gene-edited CAR T cells. Sci Transl Med 9(374)
102. Ram R, Wolach O, Vidal L, Gafter-Gvili A, Shpilberg O, Raanani P (2012) Adolescents and young adults with acute lymphoblastic leukemia have a better outcome when treated with pediatric-inspired regimens: Systematic review and meta-analysis. Am J Hematol 87:472–478
103. Roberts KG, Gu Z, Payne-Turner D et al (2017) High frequency and poor outcome of philadelphia chromosome-like acute lymphoblastic leukemia in adults. J Clin Oncol 35 (4):394–401
104. Jain N, Roberts KG, Jabbour E et al (2017) Ph-like acute lymphoblastic leukemia: a high-risk subtype in adults. Blood 129(5):572–581
105. Lacayo NJ, Pullarkat VA, Stock W et al (2019) Safety and efficacy of venetoclax in combination with navitoclax in adult and pediatric relapsed/refractory acute lymphoblastic leukemia and lymphoblastic lymphoma. Blood 134

CML Chapter

6

David Snyder

Contents

6.1 Case 1

CML, chronic phase (CP), Sokal low risk. The patient is a 29-year-old woman who was found to have a leukocytosis with a left shift on routine employment physical. She was in otherwise good health with no significant medical history. She was recently married and was interested in starting a family. She was diagnosed with CML in CP based on peripheral blood and bone marrow (BM) findings. The Ph was detected in all metaphases and polymerase chain reaction (PCR) for BCR–ABL gene using International Scale (IS) was positive at 104%. She was low risk by Sokal score. After a brief course of therapy with hydroxyurea and allopurinol, she was started on nilotinib 300 mg twice daily. Baseline EKG was normal and a repeat

D. Snyder (✉)
City of Hope Medical Center, 1500 E Duarte Rd., Duarte, CA 91010, USA
e-mail: dsnyder@coh.org

© Springer Nature Switzerland AG 2021
V. Pullarkat and G. Marcucci (eds.), *Biology and Treatment of Leukemia and Bone Marrow Neoplasms*, Cancer Treatment and Research 181,
https://doi.org/10.1007/978-3-030-78311-2_6

EKG a week after starting the nilotinib showed no prolongation of the QTc interval. She was seen every few weeks for the first few months on treatment to monitor blood counts and liver function tests. The next PCR for BCR–ABL was checked after 3 months on nilotinib. The result was 8.4552%, which met the targeted level of 10% or below by 3 months on TKIs therapy. PCR for BCR–ABL was followed every 3 months and she achieved a level of Major Molecular Response (MMR) or MR 3 by 9 months, and by 15 months on therapy, PCR became undetectable, meaning it was below MR 4.5, or 0.0032%. PCR's were monitored every 3 months and the PCR continued to be undetectable. The patient wanted to know when she could safely attempt to get pregnant and how she should manage her TKI therapy before, during, and after pregnancy.

6.2 Discussion

Several issues are raised by this case including:

Why do a BM biopsy at the time of diagnosis? The NCCN does recommend BM biopsy as part of the initial diagnostic workup, in part to be able to complete a full karyotyping study looking for the Ph and possibly other additional chromosomal aberrations. In addition, accurate staging of the disease depends on bone marrow biopsy findings since there may be signs of acceleration or blast crisis in the bone marrow that are not evident in the peripheral blood [3].

Why do PCR at the time of diagnosis? PCR for BCR–ABL is not required for diagnosis as long as the Ph is detectable by karyotyping or FISH. About 5% of patients will be Philadelphia chromosome-negative by karyotyping but BCR–ABL will be detectable either by FISH or by PCR assay. About 2% of patients may have a variant BCR–ABL transcript, for example, e13a3 [4], rather than the usual p210 transcripts of either e13a2 or e14a2. Such variant transcripts would not be detectable by standard PCR assays, and therefore the patient could not be followed in a standard lab by serial PCR assays to monitor molecular response.

On average, the PCR level for BCR–ABL in a population of patients newly diagnosed with CML will be 100% by IS [5, 6]. In actuality, there may be a wide range of PCR results at diagnosis ranging from 25 to 400% or higher. The level of PCR may be somewhat dependent on the choice of control gene that is used to calculate the ratio of BCR–ABL to a standardized gene. Most labs will use normal ABL or BCR as a control gene. Others have chosen to use a housekeeping gene unrelated to BCR or ABL as the control. As discussed below, the first goal of therapy is to reach a PCR level of 10% or below by 3 months and no later than 6 months on therapy with TKIs [7–9]. There are studies suggesting that the halving time of the PCR within 3 months based on the actual starting level of PCR may be a more accurate reflection of optimal response. Thus it may be important to determine PCR level at diagnosis to be sure the patient has a standard BCR ABL transcript and to establish the actual level of BCR–ABL gene expression by PCR at the time of diagnosis [10, 11].

Why calculate Sokal score? Sokal score was originally developed to predict responses of patients with CML to interferon [12]. The ELN has posted a website to calculate the Sokal and Hasford scores very readily (www.leukemia-net.org/content/leukemias/cml/euro__and_sokal_score/index_eng.html) It was initially unclear whether it would be of value in managing patients in the TKI era. As discussed below, the Sokal score is of value in choosing first-line therapy for newly diagnosed patients. In addition, Sokal score at diagnosis may help predict the likelihood of success when drug discontinuation is attempted in the future once the patient has achieved a deep molecular response. There are several other risks calculating systems in use such as Hasford [13] and EUTOS [14, 15] which may also be of value.

Choice of first-line TKI—first-generation vs second-generation TKI. Currently, there are four FDA approved TKIs for first-line therapy: the first-generation TKI imatinib, and second-generation TKIs dasatinib, nilotinib, and bosutinib. Based on the results of the DASISION [16], ENESTnd [17] and BFORE [18] trials, the NCCN has recommended that second-generation TKIs be chosen as first-line therapy for patients in the chronic phase who are intermediate or high risk by Sokal or Hasford score (see Table 6.1). In those trials, there were fewer cases of disease progression to accelerated phase/blast crisis in the patients who received second-generation TKIs compared to imatinib. All of those events occurred in patients who were intermediate or high risk. For patients who were low risk, the incidence of progression was very low in both first- and second-generation TKIs groups. Imatinib could be an appropriate choice as first-line therapy for patients in chronic phase, low risk, especially if they are older with associated comorbidities

Table 6.1 First-line TKI therapy for CP-CML: long-term follow-up data from phase III studies

Trial	Study Arms	N	Median Follow-Up	CCyR[a]	MMR[b]	Disease Progression, n (%)	PFS Rate[c]	OS Rate[c]
IRIS[d,39]	Imatinib (400 mg qd)	553	11 y	83%	—	38 (7%)	92%	83%
	Interferon-alpha plus low-dose cytarabine	553		—	—	71 (13%)	—	79%[e]
DASISION[40]	Dasatinib (100 mg qd)	259	5 y	—	76% (P=.002)	12 (5%)	85%	91%
	Imatinib (400 mg qd)	260		—	64%	19 (7%)	86%	90%
ENESTnd[41]	Nilotinib (300 mg bid)	282	5 y	—	77% (P vs imatinib <.0001)	10 (4%)	92%	94%
	Nilotinib (400 mg bid)	281		—	77% (P vs imatinib <.0001)	6 (2%)	96%	96%
	Imatinib (400 mg qd)	283		—	60%	21 (7%)	91%	92%
BFORE[f,42]	Bosutinib (400 mg qd)	268	12 mo	77% (P=.0075)	47% (P=.02)	4 (2%)	—	—
	Imatinib (400 mg qd)	268		66%	37%	6 (3%)	—	—

Abbreviations: CCyR, complete cytogenetic response; CP-CML, chronic phase chronic myeloid leukemia; IS, International Scale; MMR, major molecular response (BCR-ABL1 ≤0.1% IS); OS, overall survival; PFS, progression-free survival; TKI, tyrosine kinase inhibitor.
[a]Primary end point of DASISION study: confirmed CCyR rate at 12 mo.
[b]Primary end point of ENESTnd and BFORE studies: MMR (BCR-ABL1 ≤0.1%) rate at 12 mo.
[c]Long-term primary end point of IRIS trial in the imatinib group.
[d]Due to the high rate of crossover to imatinib (66%) and the short duration of therapy (<1 y) before crossover among patients who had been randomly assigned to interferon alfa plus cytarabine, the long-term follow-up data focused on patients who had been randomly assigned to receive imatinib.
[e]Data include survival among the 363 patients who crossed over to imatinib.
[f]There were no differences in survival rates between the 2 treatment arms after a minimum follow of 12 months; long term follow up is ongoing.

Table 6.2 Adverse events of first-line TKI therapy in CP-CML

Table 4. Adverse Events of First-Line TKI Therapy in CP-CML						
	DASISION[40]		ENESTnd[41]		BFORE[42]	
Toxicity	Dasatinib, 100 mg qd	Imatinib, 400 mg qd	Nilotinib, 300 mg bid	Imatinib, 400 mg qd	Bosutinib, 400 mg qd	Imatinib, 400 mg qd
Hematologic toxicities (grade 3/4)						
Anemia	13%	9%	4%	6%	3%	5%
Neutropenia	29%	24%	12%	22%	7%	12%
Thrombocytopenia	22%	14%	10%	9%	14%	6%
Biochemical abnormalities (grade 3/4)						
Increased lipase	NR	NR	9%	4%	13%	6%
Increased glucose	NR	NR	7%	<1%	2%	2%
Decreased phosphate	7%	28%	8%	10%	5%	17%
Increased ALT	NR	NR	4%	2%	23%	3%
Increased AST	NR	NR	NR	NR	12%	3%
Nonhematologic toxicities (any grade)[a]						
Rash	13%	18%	38%	19%	20%	13%
Headache	13%	11%	32%	23%	19%	13%
Fatigue	9%	11%	23%	20%	19%	18%
Muscle spasms	23%	41%	12%	34%	2%	26%
Peripheral edema	13%	37%	9%	20%	4%	14%
Pleural effusion	28%	<1%	2%	1%	NR	NR
Hypertension	NR	NR	10%	4%	NR	NR
Pulmonary hypertension	5%	<1%	0%	0%	NR	NR
Diarrhea	21%	22%	19%	46%	70%	34%
Constipation	NR	NR	20%	8%	NR	NR
Nausea	10%	24%	22%	41%	35%	39%
Vomiting	5%	11%	15%	27%	18%	16%

Abbreviations: ALT, alanine amino transferase; AST, aspartate amino transferase; CP-CML, chronic phase chronic myeloid leukemia; NR, not reported; TKI, tyrosine kinase inhibitor.
[a]Nonhematologic toxicities reported for the DASISION study (except pleural effusion) are from the 3-y follow-up. No new adverse events were observed with 5-y follow-up.

such as cardiovascular or thromboembolic disease, and if drug discontinuation is not a priority. Generic imatinib is the only available generic TKI and, generally, this is a less expensive alternative to the brand name drug, which may influence the choice of first-line TKI, especially for the insurance company if not for the patient directly. On the other hand, for a patient such as in this case, even though she is low risk, she is definitely interested in drug discontinuation and pregnancy. It is recommended that such a patient use a second-generation TKIs because these drugs are more potent than imatinib, and are likely to be more successful in achieving a deep molecular response (DMR) rapidly (see Table 6.2).

Goals of TKI therapy. The initial goals are to achieve a complete hematologic remission by 3 weeks–3 months, and a CCyR (equivalent to <=1% BCR–ABL IS) within 12 months after the start of TKI therapy. Several studies have demonstrated the importance of achieving a 3 month PCR of 10% or below. Patients who achieved this target have a high likelihood of ultimately achieving MMR by 12 months, and have superior progression-free survival. Some investigators have argued that waiting for 6 months on therapy is reasonable and that patients should not be considered to be failing unless they are still above 10% by 6 months [6–8]. Failure to achieve this level of response by 3 or possibly 6 months will generally require a change in TKI therapy to a different agent, for example. from imatinib to a second-generation TKI, or from one second-generation TKI to another. This might be an indication to check for ABL kinase domain mutations to potentially guide the choice of the next TKI based on informative mutations if present.

In the pre-TKIs era, CML patients were treated with alpha-interferon with or without cytarabine, and the main goal of therapy was to achieve CCyR. Such patients had improvement in progression-free survival. In the post TKIs era with the use of PCR monitoring, MMR or MR 3 (equivalent to 0.1% or less by PCR) has become an important goal of therapy. Patients who achieve CCyR with MMR are less likely to progress compared to patients who achieve CCyR without MMR. For the majority of patients, achievement of MMR is an appropriate goal for therapy with TKIs and it is not necessary to increase the dose of TKI or change to a more potent drug in an effort to achieve a deeper response than that [19-21].

NCCN has defined desired milestones on therapy as follows: PCR of less than 10% by 3 or 6 months; PCR less than 1% by 9 or 12 months; and PCR less than 0.1% at any time. Responses that would be of concern and require careful evaluation of issues such as patient adherence to the regimen, possible drug–drug interactions, and the need for mutational analysis include PCR greater than 10% at 6 months and PCR greater than 1% at 12 months on therapy [3].

ELN has defined optimal response as PCR less than or equal to 10% and/or Philadelphia chromosome less than or equal to 35% by 3 months; BCR–ABL less than 1% and/or undetectable Philadelphia Chromosome by 6 months; PCR less than or equal to 0.1% by 12 months. ELN has also defined response criteria for warning and failure at these time points [22].

Drug discontinuation. For some patients such as young females interested in pregnancy, or others who continue to experience ongoing low-grade toxicities from the TKIs, or for whom the financial burden of long-term therapy with TKIs is prohibitive, then the goal of achieving a DMR with the potential for drug discontinuation becomes an imperative. Several studies have been conducted looking at success rates for maintaining treatment-free remission (TFR) after drug discontinuation. Initial studies with imatinib suggested about a 50% success rate for patients who were on TKI therapy for at least 4 years in total and who were in DMR for at least 2 years [23-25]. More recent studies were conducted for patients who achieved DMR with dasatinib or nilotinib, whether as first-line or second-line therapy. The expectation was that since these TKIs are more potent than imatinib, then patients might develop even deeper molecular remissions compared to imatinib, and would have a higher success rate in maintaining TFR after drug discontinuation. However, the recent discontinuation trials with second-generation TKIs have shown almost identical TFR rates of about 50% for both dasatinib [26, 27] and nilotinib similar to the results with imatinib. Further analysis of the imatinib discontinuation studies has revealed that for patients who are treated with TKIs for a total of at least 5.8 years or longer and are in DMR for at least 3 years, they may have at least a 75% chance or higher of maintaining TFR. Other risk factors that predict for successful TFR include Sokal low risk at diagnosis, a history of meeting milestones of optimal responses to first-line TKI, and no history of progression to the accelerated phase of blast crisis or development of resistance with detection of a kinase domain mutation [28].

6.3 Case 2

Resistance to first-line TKI therapy. A 54-year-old man was diagnosed with CML, CP, Sokal intermediate risk. PCR for BCR–ABL at presentation was 120%. He was started on dasatinib 100 mg a day. The patient achieved a PCR of 9% by 3 months, but at 6–9 months was still above 1%. At 12 months, PCR increased to 15%. ABL kinase domain mutation analysis revealed the presence of T315I mutation. He was switched to ponatinib 30 mg a day. The possible need for an allogeneic hematopoietic cell transplant (HCT) was discussed with the patient. HLA typing was done on the patient and available siblings. Unrelated donor (URD) search was then carried out because no matched siblings were identified. Two 10/10 matched unrelated donors were identified. The PCR was monitored every 3 months with levels of 2, 0.6, 0.03% after 3, 6 and 9 months on ponatinib therapy. MMR was achieved and maintained over the next several years. Allogeneic HCT was not performed.

6.4 Discussion

Choice of first-line TKI. Based on ENESTnd and DASISION trials, NCCN recommends second-generation TKI as first-line therapy for CP, with intermediate or high-risk Sokal [3]. The choice of second-generation TKI may be influenced by pre-existing medical co-morbidities, patient lifestyle, and ultimately patient choice. Risks of each TKI are detailed below. For example, nilotinib must be taken twice a day with fasting for 2 hours before and 1 hour after each dose. There is a black box warning about the risk of sudden death and possible QTc prolongation. Dasatinib is taken once a day independent of food and is associated with a risk of pleural effusions. Dasatinib was chosen for this patient with an expected 5-year MMR response rate of 76% [16]. For patients who progressed on dasatinib on the DASISION trial, 10 had detectable ABL kinase domain mutations, and 7/10 of these were the T315I mutation [29]. In contrast, in the imatinib arm, there were also 10 mutations detected, but none had the T 315I mutation [30].

   Choice of second-line TKI. For patients who are intolerant of the first-line choice of TKI, any of the other three TKIs approved for first-line therapy could be chosen as second-line therapy. For patients who are resistant to the first-line choice, then BCR–ABL mutation analysis should be carried out. Such mutations will be found in up to 75% of resistant cases. If a specific mutation is identified then the choice of second-line TKI should be dictated by the known sensitivities of that mutation [31–33]. For example, mutations such as E255K and Y253H are resistant to imatinib; V299L is resistant to bosutinib and dasatinib. The T315I mutation is highly resistant to all available TKIs other than ponatinib [34–36]. This drug can be given in three doses: 15, 30, or 45 mg a day. There is a known risk of major thromboembolic events of approximately 27%. Most of these events are arterial rather than venous and occur at a higher frequency in patients who have co-morbidities such as diabetes, hypertension, and hyperlipidemia. The risk is also dependent on the dose of ponatinib. The optimal dose strategy is uncertain at this time. Risk mitigation measures call for using a lower dose from the beginning and then escalate if needed. Alternatively, one could start with 45 mg a day, and then dose reduces when the goal of MMR is achieved. Allogeneic HCT may be the only option available for patients with T315I mutation who fail to respond to or tolerate ponatinib. Omacetaxine is the only other FDA-approved drug indicated for the treatment of CML with the T315I mutation, although the response rates to this drug are lower than for ponatinib [37]. Omacetaxine is a protein synthesis inhibitor, not a TKI, and myelosuppression is a significant toxicity risk.

6.5 Case 3

CML, blast crisis (BC). A 32-year-old woman was diagnosed with CML in blast crisis based on bone marrow biopsy and lymph node biopsy. She presented to her doctor with complaints of mild headaches with tenderness and swelling along the right side of her neck starting behind the ear. She had seen a doctor about 2 years before then because she was having pain in the pelvis and she was told she had leukocytosis possibly due to infection at that time. At presentation, she had four enlarged lymph nodes with the largest just behind the right ear and three more in the cervical chain. She had splenomegaly with symptoms of early satiety. She had WBC 66.3, hemoglobin 9.5, hematocrit 30.3, platelets 604,000. Differential showed 86% segmented neutrophils and bands, 3% lymphocytes, 1% monocytes, 3% eosinophils, 4% basophils, and 2.5% blasts. She was positive for BCR–ABL by PCR and negative for JAK2 mutation. BM biopsy showed 100% cellular marrow with 3% B lymphoblasts by flow and 3.5% myeloblasts. Cytogenetics from bone marrow showed the Ph chromosome in 20/20 metaphases. There were no other cytogenetic abnormalities.

A biopsy of the right cervical lymph node showed evidence of CML with the mixed phenotype of blast crisis with cells that were positive by immunophenotyping for a variety of T-cell, B-cell, and myeloid blast markers. Cytogenetics from the lymph node were complex with Ph chromosome in all metaphases but also multiple other changes involving chromosomes 1, 3, 5, 6, 10, 15, 17p, 19, and a marker chromosome.

She started chemotherapy with hyper-CVAD cycle 1 part A and dasatinib 140 mg a day prescribed as 70 mg twice daily. Dasatinib was put on hold after a few weeks because of the cytopenias. She had a repeat bone marrow biopsy that was hypocellular at about 10% with no blasts seen. She had two lumbar punctures with intrathecal chemotherapy and both were negative for leukemia cells. She was referred to a transplant center urgently. Fortunately, her only sister was a full 10/10 HLA match. The patient was of Native Mexican ancestry with no full or partly matched donors identified in the international donor registry. She was conditioned with dose-adjusted intravenous busulfan and cyclophosphamide. She received tacrolimus and full dose methotrexate for graft versus host disease (GVHD) prophylaxis.

PCR for BCR–ABL just before transplant was 2.6401%. PCR was undetectable at the day +30 bone marrow, but on day +60 peripheral blood it was positive at 0.2627%. Her immunosuppression was reduced and she was started on dasatinib 50 mg daily. 6 weeks later the PCR was 0.0473%, and a month later it was undetectable. She then developed GVHD affecting the skin and liver with marked elevation of transaminases and alkaline phosphatase and dasatinib was put on hold. Immunosuppression was escalated to control the GVHD. Her LFTs remain elevated and dasatinib remained on hold. After several weeks, the liver tests improved, the immunosuppression was tapered down, and dasatinib was restarted at 50 mg a day.

6.6 Discussion

Management of blast crisis

Patients may present in blast crisis that is apparent in the blood and bone marrow. However, in some patients such as the patient in this case, the blood and bone marrow appear to be chronic phase, but extramedullary sites of involvement such as central nervous system or lymph nodes, demonstrate the presence of blasts [38, 39]. Blast crisis of CML may involve any lineage, most commonly myeloid or B lymphoid [40]. Rarely the T lymphoid lineage may be involved in extramedullary blast crisis of CML, [41, 42] and even more rarely there may be multiple lineages involved at the same time such as this case. Patients who present in blast crisis must go through a course of appropriate induction chemotherapy in combination with TKIs, and then proceed as soon as possible to an allogeneic stem cell transplant. This strategy is the only chance of cure for these patients. The choice of induction chemotherapy is dependent on the nature of the blasts. For myeloid blast crisis, a regimen that uses cytarabine and anthracycline, or possibly high-dose cytarabine is often recommended. For lymphoid blast crisis a standard ALL induction regimen is recommended. In this case, that involved myeloid, B-cell, and T-cell lineages, hyper-CVAD regimen was an appropriate choice [43–45].

Allogenic stem cell transplantation

There has been a dramatic decline in the number of allogeneic stem cell transplants performed for CML since the advent of TKIs. Before imatinib was approved, allogeneic stem cell transplantation was the mainstay of therapy for younger patients with newly diagnosed CML. CML was one of the most common diagnoses for which allogeneic stem cell transplantation was performed in the pre-TKIs era.

Currently, stem cell transplantation is very rarely indicated since the vast majority of patients with CML are managed successfully with one TKI or another. A small number of transplants are performed yearly for patients with CML who generally fit into one of the following three categories:

1. Patients who developed the T315I mutation and did not respond adequately to or cannot tolerate ponatinib.
2. Patients who present in blast crisis or progress to blast crisis after initial therapy with TKIs for chronic-phase disease.
3. Patients who are intolerant of or resistant to all available TKIs. In the post-TKIs era, therefore, the patients who do come to transplant are generally more refractory and advanced than the cohorts of patients who were transplanted pre-TKIs. Results from transplantation have been reported recently and confirm the importance of disease phase as an important prognostic factor for post-transplant survival. Thus, patients in CP have better outcomes than patients who are in AP or BC at the time of transplant. Other important risk factors include HLA matching, age and sex of the donor and recipient, and time from diagnosis to transplant [46–53].

In some countries in which TKIs therapy is very expensive or not readily available, an allogeneic stem cell transplant from a well-matched donor may be a reasonable strategy for young, otherwise healthy patients with newly diagnosed CML [54, 55]. Recent reports have shown over 90% disease-free survival in good risk patients reflecting the efficacy of transplant with a low acceptable complication rate [51].

Management of post-transplant relapse

Post-transplant relapse of CML is one of the known complications of this approach, especially for patients who are in the advanced stage of the disease when they come to transplant. The general practice for such patients is to preemptively or prophy-lactically reinstitute TKIs post-transplant. The optimal timing for re-starting TKIs, and the choice of TKIs post-transplant is an unsettled issue. Definite proof that this practice is effective is lacking in terms of randomized control trials. Combining TKIs with Donor Lymphocyte Infusions may offer the best chance of controlling post-transplant relapse [56–70].

6.7 Risks of TKIs

It is important to be aware of the risks associated with the various TKIs available when making a choice for first-line or salvage therapy [71] (see Table 6.3). Each patient's pre-existing comorbidities need to be assessed in light of these risks. Certain toxicities are common to all of the TKIs such as myelosuppression, elevated transaminases, electrolyte changes, QT prolongation, skin rashes, and fluid

Table 6.3 First-line TKI therapy for CP-CML: MR rates according to Sokal or Euro risk score

Table 3. First-Line TKI Therapy for CP-CML: MR Rates According to Sokal or Euro Risk Score		Low-Risk[a,b]		Intermediate-Risk[a,b]		High-Risk[a,b]	
Trial	Study Arms	MMR	MR4.5	MMR	MR4.5	MMR	MR4.5
DASISION[40]	Dasatinib (100 mg qd)	90%	55%	71%	43%	67%	31%
	Imatinib (400 mg qd)	69%	44%	65%	28%	54%	30%
ENESTnd[41]	Nilotinib (300 mg bid)	—	53%	—	60%	—	45%
	Nilotinib (400 mg bid)	—	62%	—	50%	—	42%
	Imatinib (400 mg qd)	—	38%	—	33%	—	23%
BFORE[42]	Bosutinib (400 mg qd)	58%	—	45%	—	34%	—
	Imatinib (400 mg qd)	46%	—	39%	—	17%	—

Abbreviations: CP-CML, chronic phase chronic myeloid leukemia; IS, International Scale; MMR, major molecular response (≤0.1% *BCR-ABL1* IS); MR, molecular response; MR4.5: 4.5-log reduction in *BCR-ABL1* transcripts from baseline; TKI, tyrosine kinase inhibitor.
[a]DASISION study: Risk stratification by Hasford (Euro) risk score.
[b]ENESTnd and BFORE trial: Risk stratification by Sokal risk score.

retention. In addition, each of the five FDA-approved TKIs has its own profile of toxicities that may be unique or more severe with one TKI versus another. Imatinib is associated with periorbital edema and peripheral edema, myalgias, hypophosphatemia, GI toxicity, and possible renal impairment. Nilotinib has been associated with the risk of vascular adverse events such as peripheral arterial occlusive disease, hyperglycemia, hyperlipidemia, pancreatic enzyme elevation, and indirect hyperbilirubinemia. Dasatinib has been associated with the risk of pleural and pericardial effusions, pulmonary arterial hypertension, risk of hemorrhage from the GI tract and elsewhere, and rarely reactive lymphadenopathy. Bosutinib has been associated mainly with GI toxicities such as diarrhea and nausea, elevated transaminases, and possible renal effects. Ponatinib is the most potent TKI available and has the highest risk of cardiovascular toxicity including serious thromboembolic events in up to 27% of patients including strokes, myocardial infarction, and hypertension.

For patients who have significant risk factors for thromboembolic disease, imatinib may be a safer choice for initial TKI therapy. Bosutinib is also associated with low risk of cardiovascular complications and is now approved as first-line therapy for newly diagnosed patients.

Risk mitigation strategies have been proposed to increase the safety of therapy with ponatinib. The incidence of thromboembolic events is dose-dependent and it may be advisable to initiate therapy at a lower dose, for example, 15 or 30 mg daily, and then escalate the dose only if there is a lack of efficacy. An alternative approach which is being tested in randomized phase 3 trial, would be to start patients at a higher dose, and then reduce the dose to a lower level once the desired endpoint has been achieved. It has become general practice to use low-dose aspirin in patients treated with ponatinib although there are no controlled studies to document the protective effects of aspirin in this setting. Some clinicians have suggested treating patients with a statin while on ponatinib. Careful attention to traditional risk factors such as smoking, hypertension, diabetes, and hyperlipidemia is critical. Partnering with a cardiologist or endocrinologist to manage these comorbidities is strongly advised.

6.8 Future Directions and Unmet Needs

The treatment of CML in the TKI era has been a remarkable success story. Most patients with CML can expect a near-normal life expectancy [72]. It is difficult to know how this success could be improved upon. The fact remains that the vast majority of newly diagnosed patients with CML will need to stay on TKIs lifelong. Such therapy is associated with a variety of toxicities that may impair quality of life. Patients may be overwhelmed by the financial burden of the costs of this therapy. Young women interested in having families represent a subset of patients for whom long-term therapy with TKIs is unacceptable [73, 74]. Thus there are compelling reasons to pursue novel strategies that could lead to the complete discontinuation of TKI therapy for the vast majority of patients.

It is estimated that only about 12–15% of all newly diagnosed patients with CML in chronic phase will ultimately achieve TFR. This estimate is based on the fact that about 25% of patients will achieve a sustained deep molecular remission, and of those patients, only about 50% will successfully maintain TFR after discontinuation of TKIs. The question that should be raised is not: Why is the TFR success rate only 50%, but rather: Why do any patients achieve TFR? After all, the CML leukemic stem cell is known to be resistant to the pro-apoptotic effects of TKIs [75]. The leukemic stem cells persist in a quiescent phase even in patients who achieve complete molecular remission with TKIs therapy. Presumably, the pool of leukemic stem cells should reactivate and repopulate the leukemic cell population after discontinuation of TKIs. Why then do not all patients ultimately relapse after discontinuation of TKIs?

There are two theories to explain the lack of relapse after drug discontinuation. The first is the concept of stem cell pool exhaustion which means that due to the effects of a drug, or just with the passage of time, there is gradual attrition of this population of cells based on their finite lifespan. That theory is offered as an explanation as to why the TFR success rate is higher the longer patients have been treated with TKIs from the time of diagnosis to the time of attempted drug discontinuation. Those patients who were treated with TKIs for 4 years in total have a TFR success rate of about 50%, whereas patients who are maintained on TKIs for at least 5.8 years or longer may reach success rates of 75% or higher.

A therapeutic approach to kill off leukemic stem cells would be another way to eradicate all remnants of CML and potentially cure patients. Several groups are testing the concept of combination therapy with a TKI plus a second agent that works through a completely different mechanism of action, which together may synergize to kill off the resistant leukemic stem cells or promote exhaustion of the pool. Examples of this approach include a combination of TKI with a histone deacetylase inhibitor [76]; alpha-interferon [77, 78]; miRNA inhibition [79]; a novel TKI called asciminib (ABL001) that targets the myristoyl binding site of the BCR–ABL protein [80]; and others [81–86].

The second theory to explain the lack of relapse focuses on the patient's immune response to CML stem cells. It is postulated that some components of the patient's immune system may prevent the reactivation of residual quiescent stem cells to explain the lack of relapse after drug discontinuation. Several studies have focused on the role of NK cells in this regard. There are data to suggest that patients who have increased numbers and/or increased activity of NK cells may have a higher likelihood of achieving and maintaining TFR [87, 88]. There may be other components of the immune system that are important as well. Strategies that serve to boost the patient's NK cell number and activity may be a way to increase the rate of TFR. This concept of immune surveillance and immune reactivity against residual leukemic stem cells underlies the success and curative outcomes of allogeneic stem cell transplantation. In that setting, the allo-reactive T cells from the donor are thought to be responsible for the prevention of reactivation of residual quiescent leukemic stem cells long term.

There is a novel agent under study called Asciminib (ABL001) which is a BCR–ABL1 inhibitor distinct from approved TKIs in that it does not bind to the ATP-binding site of the kinase. Rather asciminib acts as an allosteric inhibitor and engages a vacant pocket at a site of the kinase domain normally occupied by the myristoylated N-terminal of ABL1—a motif that serves as an allosteric negative regulatory element lost on the fusion of ABL1 to BCR. This drug showed activity in CML patients who had failed previous TKI therapy, even for those with the T315I mutation [89]. In the future, combination therapy with asciminib plus a TKI may be an effective strategy for treating newly diagnosed patients.

Disease progression from chronic phase to accelerated phase or blast crisis is still a significant problem for the minority of patients who failed to achieve adequate responses to TKIs therapy. Strategies to identify those patients at risk for progression at an earlier time point would be of value. Molecular profiling of patients to detect additional molecular mutations besides BCR–ABL, may help with this goal. Combining a TKI with a second agent that works through a different mechanism of action which might synergize with the TKI might be an effective strategy to help prevent progression.

Taking a global perspective, it is clear that a large portion of the developing world is unable to benefit from the breakthroughs and diagnostic and therapeutic options available for patients with CML. Doctors in these countries have very little limited resources to be able to diagnose and monitor CML because of the technical requirements and expense of PCR assays. Treatment of patients is limited by the huge expense of TKIs and by the limited number of agents that are available in many countries. Imatinib may be the only option available so that for patients who progress on imatinib, the only option is to increase the dose of the drug until a maximum tolerated dose. Beyond that such patients have no real options. Organizations such as the iCMLf and Max Foundation are working to try to overcome some of these barriers.

References

1. Hochhaus A, Larson RA, Guilhot F, Radich JP, Branford S, Hughes TP et al (2017) Long-term outcomes of imatinib treatment for chronic myeloid leukemia. N Engl J Med 376 (10):917–927
2. Soverini S, Mancini M, Bavaro L, Cavo M, Martinelli G (2018) Chronic myeloid leukemia: the paradigm of targeting oncogenic tyrosine kinase signaling and counteracting resistance for successful cancer therapy. Mol Cancer 17(1):49
3. Radich JP, Deininger M, Abboud CN, Altman JK, Berman E, Bhatia R et al (2018) Chronic myeloid leukemia, Version 1.2019, NCCN clinical practice guidelines in oncology. J Natl Comprehensive Cancer Netw 16(9):1108–1135
4. Snyder DS, McMahon R, Cohen SR, Slovak ML (2004) Chronic myeloid leukemia with an e13a3 BCR-ABL fusion: benign course responsive to imatinib with an RT-PCR advisory. Am J Hematol 75(2):92–95
5. Cross NC (2009) Standardisation of molecular monitoring for chronic myeloid leukaemia. Best Pract Res Clin Haematol 22(3):355–365
6. Branford S, Cross NC, Hochhaus A, Radich J, Saglio G, Kaeda J et al (2006) Rationale for the recommendations for harmonizing current methodology for detecting BCR-ABL transcripts in patients with chronic myeloid leukaemia. Leukemia 20(11):1925–1930
7. Hanfstein B, Muller MC, Hehlmann R, Erben P, Lauseker M, Fabarius A et al (2012) Early molecular and cytogenetic response is predictive for long-term progression-free and overall survival in chronic myeloid leukemia (CML). Leukemia 26(9):2096–2102
8. Marin D, Ibrahim AR, Lucas C, Gerrard G, Wang L, Szydlo RM et al (2012) Assessment of BCR-ABL1 transcript levels at 3 months is the only requirement for predicting outcome for patients with chronic myeloid leukemia treated with tyrosine kinase inhibitors. J Clin Oncol 30(3):232–238
9. Nazha A, Kantarjian H, Jain P, Romo C, Jabbour E, Quintas-Cardama A et al (2013) Assessment at 6 months may be warranted for patients with chronic myeloid leukemia with no major cytogenetic response at 3 months. Haematologica 98(11):1686–1688
10. Hanfstein B, Shlyakhto V, Lauseker M, Hehlmann R, Saussele S, Dietz C et al (2014) Velocity of early BCR-ABL transcript elimination as an optimized predictor of outcome in chronic myeloid leukemia (CML) patients in chronic phase on treatment with imatinib. Leukemia 28(10):1988–1992
11. Iriyama N, Fujisawa S, Yoshida C, Wakita H, Chiba S, Okamoto S et al (2015) Shorter halving time of BCR-ABL1 transcripts is a novel predictor for achievement of molecular responses in newly diagnosed chronic-phase chronic myeloid leukemia treated with dasatinib: results of the D-first study of Kanto CML study group. Am J Hematol 90(4):282–287
12. Sokal JE, Cox EB, Baccarani M, Tura S, Gomez GA, Robertson JE et al (1984) Prognostic discrimination in "good-risk" chronic granulocytic leukemia. Blood 63(4):789–799
13. Hasford J, Pfirrmann M, Hehlmann R, Allan NC, Baccarani M, Kluin-Nelemans JC et al (1998) A new prognostic score for survival of patients with chronic myeloid leukemia treated with interferon alfa. J Natl Cancer Inst 90(11):850–858
14. Jabbour E, Cortes J, Nazha A, O'Brien S, Quintas-Cardama A, Pierce S et al (2012) EUTOS score is not predictive for survival and outcome in patients with early chronic phase chronic myeloid leukemia treated with tyrosine kinase inhibitors: a single institution experience. Blood 119(19):4524–4526
15. Uz B, Buyukasik Y, Atay H, Kelkitli E, Turgut M, Bektas O et al (2013) EUTOS CML prognostic scoring system predicts ELN-based 'event-free survival' better than Euro/Hasford and Sokal systems in CML patients receiving front-line imatinib mesylate. Hematology 18 (5):247–252
16. Cortes JE, Saglio G, Kantarjian HM, Baccarani M, Mayer J, Boqué C et al (2016) Final 5-year study results of dasision: the dasatinib versus imatinib study in treatment-naïve chronic myeloid leukemia patients trial. J Clin Oncol 34(20):2333–2340

17. Hochhaus A, Saglio G, Hughes TP, Larson RA, Kim DW, Issaragrisil S et al (2016) Long-term benefits and risks of frontline nilotinib vs imatinib for chronic myeloid leukemia in chronic phase: 5-year update of the randomized ENESTnd trial. Leukemia 30(5):1044–1054

18. Cortes JE, Gambacorti-Passerini C, Deininger MW, Mauro MJ, Chuah C, Kim DW et al (2018) Bosutinib versus imatinib for newly diagnosed chronic myeloid leukemia: results from the randomized bfore trial. J Clin Oncol 36(3):231–237

19. Hughes TP, Hochhaus A, Branford S, Muller MC, Kaeda JS, Foroni L et al (2010) Long-term prognostic significance of early molecular response to imatinib in newly diagnosed chronic myeloid leukemia: an analysis from the international randomized study of interferon and STI571 (IRIS). Blood 116(19):3758–3765

20. Druker BJ, Guilhot F, O'Brien SG, Gathmann I, Kantarjian H, Gattermann N et al (2006) Five-year follow-up of patients receiving imatinib for chronic myeloid leukemia. N Engl J Med 355(23):2408–2417

21. Marin D, Milojkovic D, Olavarria E, Khorashad JS, de Lavallade H, Reid AG et al (2008) European LeukemiaNet criteria for failure or suboptimal response reliably identify patients with CML in early chronic phase treated with imatinib whose eventual outcome is poor. Blood 112(12):4437–4444

22. Baccarani M, Deininger MW, Rosti G, Hochhaus A, Soverini S, Apperley JF et al (2013) European LeukemiaNet recommendations for the management of chronic myeloid leukemia: 2013. Blood 122(6):872–884

23. Mahon FX, Rea D, Guilhot J, Guilhot F, Huguet F, Nicolini F et al (2010) Discontinuation of imatinib in patients with chronic myeloid leukaemia who have maintained complete molecular remission for at least 2 years: the prospective, multicentre Stop Imatinib (STIM) trial. Lancet Oncol 11(11):1029–1035

24. Etienne G, Guilhot J, Rea D, Rigal-Huguet F, Nicolini F, Charbonnier A et al (2017) Long-term follow-up of the french stop imatinib (STIM1) study in patients with chronic myeloid leukemia. J Clin Oncol 35(3):298–305

25. Rousselot P, Charbonnier A, Cony-Makhoul P, Agape P, Nicolini FE, Varet B et al (2014) Loss of major molecular response as a trigger for restarting tyrosine kinase inhibitor therapy in patients with chronic-phase chronic myelogenous leukemia who have stopped imatinib after durable undetectable disease. J Clin Oncol 32(5):424–430

26. Ross DM, Masszi T, Gomez Casares MT, Hellmann A, Stentoft J, Conneally E et al (2018) Durable treatment-free remission in patients with chronic myeloid leukemia in chronic phase following frontline nilotinib: 96-week update of the ENESTfreedom study. J Cancer Res Clin Oncol 144(5):945–954

27. Okada M, Imagawa J, Tanaka H, Nakamae H, Hino M, Murai K et al (2018) Final 3-year results of the dasatinib discontinuation trial in patients with chronic myeloid leukemia who received dasatinib as a second-line treatment. Clin Lymphoma, Myeloma Leukemia 18 (5):353–360 e1

28. Rousselot P (2018) The story of tyrosine kinase inhibitors discontinuation in clinical practice. Leuk Lymphoma 1–10

29. Chan W, Wise S, Kaufman M, Ahn Y, Ensinger C, Haack T et al (2011) Conformational control inhibition of the BCR-ABL1 tyrosine kinase, including the gatekeeper T315I mutant, by the switch-control inhibitor DCC-2036. Cancer Cell 19(4):556–568

30. Kantarjian HM, Shah NP, Cortes JE, Baccarani M, Agarwal MB, Undurraga MaS et al (2012) Dasatinib or imatinib in newly diagnosed chronic-phase chronic myeloid leukemia: 2-year follow-up from a randomized phase 3 trial (DASISION). Blood 119(5):1123–1129

31. Cortes JE, Khoury HJ, Kantarjian HM, Lipton JH, Kim D-W, Schafhausen P et al (2016) Long-term bosutinib for chronic phase chronic myeloid leukemia after failure of imatinib plus dasatinib and/or nilotinib. Am J Hematol 91(12):1206–1214

32. Giles FJ, le Coutre PD, Pinilla-Ibarz J, Larson RA, Gattermann N, Ottmann OG et al (2013) Nilotinib in imatinib-resistant or imatinib-intolerant patients with chronic myeloid leukemia in chronic phase: 48-month follow-up results of a phase II study. Leukemia 27(1):107–112

33. Shah NP, Rousselot P, Schiffer C, Rea D, Cortes JE, Milone J et al (2016) Dasatinib in imatinib-resistant or -intolerant chronic-phase, chronic myeloid leukemia patients: 7-year follow-up of study CA180-034. Am J Hematol 91(9):869–874

34. Cortes JE, Kim DW, Pinilla-Ibarz J, le Coutre PD, Paquette R, Chuah C et al (2018) Ponatinib efficacy and safety in Philadelphia chromosome-positive leukemia: final 5-year results of the phase 2 PACE trial. Blood 132(4):393–404

35. Jabbour E, Kantarjian H, Jones D, Breeden M, Garcia-Manero G, O'Brien S et al (2008) Characteristics and outcomes of patients with chronic myeloid leukemia and T315I mutation following failure of imatinib mesylate therapy. Blood 112(1):53–55

36. Nicolini FE, Hayette S, Corm S, Bachy E, Bories D, Tulliez M et al (2007) Clinical outcome of 27 imatinib mesylate-resistant chronic myelogenous leukemia patients harboring a T315I BCR-ABL mutation. Haematologica 92(9):1238–1241

37. Khoury HJ, Cortes J, Baccarani M, Wetzler M, Masszi T, Digumarti R et al (2015) Omacetaxine mepesuccinate in patients with advanced chronic myeloid leukemia with resistance or intolerance to tyrosine kinase inhibitors. Leuk Lymphoma 56(1):120–127

38. Calabretta B, Perrotti D (2004) The biology of CML blast crisis. Blood 103(11):4010–4022

39. Specchia G, Palumbo G, Pastore D, Mininni D, Mestice A, Liso V (1996) Extramedullary blast crisis in chronic myeloid leukemia. LeukRes. 20:905–908

40. Urbano-Ispizua A, Cervantes F, Matutes E, Villamor N, Pujades A, Sierra J et al (1993) Immunophenotypic characteristics of blast crisis of chronic myeloid leukaemia: correlations with clinico-biological features and survival. Leukemia 7:1349–1354

41. Ye CC, Echeverri C, Anderson JE, Smith JL, Glassman A, Gulley ML et al (2002) T-celL blast crisis of chronic myelogenous leukemia manifesting as a large mediastinal tumor. Hum Pathol 33(7):770–773

42. Lucero G, Birman V, Colimodio E, Bertinetti CM, Kotliar N, Murolo P et al (2000) Nodal T cell blast crisis in chronic myeloid leukemia. Leuk Lymphoma 39(3–4):435–440

43. Strati P, Kantarjian H, Thomas D, O'Brien S, Konoplev S, Jorgensen JL et al (2014) HCVAD plus imatinib or dasatinib in lymphoid blastic phase chronic myeloid leukemia. Cancer 120 (3):373–380

44. Radich J (2016) When to consider allogeneic transplantation in CML. Clin Lymphoma Myeloma Leuk 16(Suppl):S93–S95

45. Hehlmann R (2012) How I treat CML blast crisis. Blood 120(4):737–747

46. Boehm A, Walcherberger B, Sperr WR, Wohrer S, Dieckmann K, Rosenmayr A et al (2011) Improved outcome in patients with chronic myelogenous leukemia after allogeneic hematopoietic stem cell transplantation over the past 25 years: a single-center experience. Biol Blood Marrow Transplant: J Am Soc Blood Marrow Transplant 17(1):133–140

47. Jabbour E, Cortes J, Santos FP, Jones D, O'Brien S, Rondon G et al (2011) Results of allogeneic hematopoietic stem cell transplantation for chronic myelogenous leukemia patients who failed tyrosine kinase inhibitors after developing BCR-ABL1 kinase domain mutations. Blood 117(13):3641–3647

48. Khoury HJ, Kukreja M, Goldman JM, Wang T, Halter J, Arora M et al (2012) Prognostic factors for outcomes in allogeneic transplantation for CML in the imatinib era: a CIBMTR analysis. Bone Marrow Transplant 47(6):810–816

49. Lee SE, Choi SY, Kim SH, Jang EJ, Bang JH, Byeun JY et al (2014) Prognostic factors for outcomes of allogeneic stem cell transplantation in chronic phase chronic myeloid leukemia in the era of tyrosine kinase inhibitors. Hematology 19(2):63–72

50. Nicolini FE, Basak GW, Kim DW, Olavarria E, Pinilla-Ibarz J, Apperley JF et al (2017) Overall survival with ponatinib versus allogeneic stem cell transplantation in Philadelphia chromosome-positive leukemias with the T315I mutation. Cancer 123(15):2875–2880

51. Saussele S, Lauseker M, Gratwohl A, Beelen DW, Bunjes D, Schwerdtfeger R et al (2010) Allogeneic hematopoietic stem cell transplantation (allo SCT) for chronic myeloid leukemia in the imatinib era: evaluation of its impact within a subgroup of the randomized German CML study IV. Blood 115(10):1880–1885

52. Warlick E, Ahn KW, Pedersen TL, Artz A, de Lima M, Pulsipher M et al (2012) Reduced intensity conditioning is superior to nonmyeloablative conditioning for older chronic myelogenous leukemia patients undergoing hematopoietic cell transplant during the tyrosine kinase inhibitor era. Blood 119(17):4083–4090

53. Nair AP, Barnett MJ, Broady RC, Hogge DE, Song KW, Toze CL et al (2015) Allogeneic hematopoietic stem cell transplantation is an effective salvage therapy for patients with chronic myeloid leukemia presenting with advanced disease or failing treatment with tyrosine kinase inhibitors. Biol Blood Marrow Transplant: J Am Soc Blood Marrow Transplant 21 (8):1437–1444

54. Zheng C, Zhu X, Tang B, Zhang X, Zhang L, Geng L et al (2018) Transplants of unrelated cord blood or sibling allogeneic peripheral blood stem cells/bone marrow in adolescent and young adults with chronic myeloid leukemia: comparable outcomes but better chronic GVHD-free and relapse-free survival among survivors with cord blood. Oncotarget 9 (2):2848–2857

55. Pasquini MC (2012) Hematopoietic cell transplantation for chronic myeloid leukemia in developing countries: perspectives from Latin America in the post-tyrosine kinase inhibitor era. Hematology 17(Suppl 1):S79-82

56. Zeidner JF, Zahurak M, Rosner GL, Gocke CD, Jones RJ, Smith BD (2015) The evolution of treatment strategies for patients with chronic myeloid leukemia relapsing after allogeneic bone marrow transplant: can tyrosine kinase inhibitors replace donor lymphocyte infusions? Leuk Lymphoma 56(1):128–134

57. Shanavas M, Messner HA, Kamel-Reid S, Atenafu EG, Gupta V, Kuruvilla J et al (2014) A comparison of long-term outcomes of donor lymphocyte infusions and tyrosine kinase inhibitors in patients with relapsed CML after allogeneic hematopoietic cell transplantation. Clin Lymphoma Myeloma Leuk 14(1):87–92

58. DeFilipp Z, Langston AA, Chen Z, Zhang C, Arellano ML, El Rassi F et al (2016) Does post-transplant maintenance therapy with tyrosine kinase inhibitors improve outcomes of patients with high-risk philadelphia chromosome-positive leukemia? Clin Lymphoma Myeloma Leuk 16(8):466–71.e1

59. Chalandon Y, Iacobelli S, Hoek J, Koster L, Volin L, Finke J et al (2016) Use of first or second generation TKI for CML after allogeneic stem cell transplantation: a study by the CMWP of the EBMT. Blood 128(22):4685

60. Egan DN, Beppu L, Radich JP (2015) Patients with Philadelphia-positive leukemia with BCR-ABL kinase mutations before allogeneic transplantation predominantly relapse with the same mutation. Biol Blood Marrow Transplant: J Am Soc Blood Marrow Transplant 21 (1):184–189

61. Anderlini P, Sheth S, Hicks K, Ippoliti C, Giralt S, Champlin RE (2004) Re: Imatinib mesylate administration in the first 100 days after stem cell transplantation. Biol Blood Marrow Transplant: J Am Soc Blood Marrow Transplant 10(12):883–884

62. DeAngelo DJ, Hochberg EP, Alyea EP, Longtine J, Lee S, Galinsky I et al (2004) Extended follow-up of patients treated with imatinib mesylate (gleevec) for chronic myelogenous leukemia relapse after allogeneic transplantation: durable cytogenetic remission and conversion to complete donor chimerism without graft-versus-host disease. Clin Cancer Res 10(15):5065–5071

63. Hess G, Bunjes D, Siegert W, Schwerdtfeger R, Ledderose G, Wassmann B et al (2005) Sustained complete molecular remissions after treatment with imatinib-mesylate in patients with failure after allogeneic stem cell transplantation for chronic myelogenous leukemia: results of a prospective phase II open-label multicenter study. J Clin Oncol 23(30):7583–7593

64. Shimoni A, Volchek Y, Koren-Michowitz M, Varda-Bloom N, Somech R, Shem-Tov N et al (2015) Phase 1/2 study of nilotinib prophylaxis after allogeneic stem cell transplantation in patients with advanced chronic myeloid leukemia or Philadelphia chromosome-positive acute lymphoblastic leukemia. Cancer 121(6):863–871

65. Klyuchnikov E, Schafhausen P, Kroger N, Brummendorf TH, Osanmaz O, Asenova S et al (2009) Second-generation tyrosine kinase inhibitors in the post-transplant period in patients with chronic myeloid leukemia or Philadelphia-positive acute lymphoblastic leukemia. Acta Haematol 122(1):6–10

66. Carpenter PA, Snyder DS, Flowers ME, Sanders JE, Gooley TA, Martin PJ et al (2007) Prophylactic administration of imatinib after hematopoietic cell transplantation for high-risk Philadelphia chromosome-positive leukemia. Blood 109(7):2791–2793

67. Carpenter PA, Johnston L, Fernandez HF, Radich JP, Mauro MJ, Flowers MED et al (2017) Posttransplant feasibility study of nilotinib prophylaxis for high-risk Philadelphia chromosome positive leukemia. Blood 130(9):1170–1172

68. Olavarria E, Siddique S, Griffiths MJ, Avery S, Byrne JL, Piper KP et al (2007) Posttransplantation imatinib as a strategy to postpone the requirement for immunotherapy in patients undergoing reduced-intensity allografts for chronic myeloid leukemia. Blood 110 (13):4614–4617

69. Wright MP, Shepherd JD, Barnett MJ, Nantel SH, Sutherland HJ, Toze CL et al (2010) Response to tyrosine kinase inhibitor therapy in patients with chronic myelogenous leukemia relapsing in chronic and advanced phase following allogeneic hematopoietic stem cell transplantation. Biol Blood Marrow Transplant: J Am Soc Blood Marrow Transplant 16 (5):639–646

70. Palandri F, Amabile M, Rosti G, Bandini G, Benedetti F, Usala E et al (2007) Imatinib therapy for chronic myeloid leukemia patients who relapse after allogeneic stem cell transplantation: a molecular analysis. Bone Marrow Transplant 39(3):189–191

71. Kennedy JA, Hobbs G (2018) Tyrosine kinase inhibitors in the treatment of chronic-phase cml: strategies for frontline decision-making. Curr Hematol Malig Rep 13(3):202–211

72. Bower H, Bjorkholm M, Dickman PW, Hoglund M, Lambert PC, Andersson TM (2016) Life expectancy of patients with chronic myeloid leukemia approaches the life expectancy of the general population. J Clin Oncol 34(24):2851–2857

73. Law AD, Dong Hwan Kim D, Lipton JH (2017) Pregnancy: part of life in chronic myelogenous leukemia. Leuk Lymphoma 58(2):280–287

74. Cortes JE, Abruzzese E, Chelysheva E, Guha M, Wallis N, Apperley JF (2015) The impact of dasatinib on pregnancy outcomes. Am J Hematol 90(12):1111–1115

75. Moreno-Lorenzana D, Aviles-Vazquez S, Sandoval Esquivel MA, Alvarado-Moreno A, Ortiz-Navarrete V, Torres-Martinez H et al (2016) CDKIs p18(INK4c) and p57(Kip2) are involved in quiescence of CML leukemic stem cells after treatment with TKI. Cell Cycle (Georgetown, Tex). 15(9):1276–1287

76. Zhang B, Strauss AC, Chu S, Li M, Ho Y, Shiang KD et al (2010) Effective targeting of quiescent chronic myelogenous leukemia stem cells by histone deacetylase inhibitors in combination with imatinib mesylate. Cancer Cell 17(5):427–442

77. Yokota A, Hirai H, Hayashi Y, Sato R, Adachi H, Sato F et al (2016) C/EBPβ is a critical regulator of CML stem cell differentiation and exhaustion induced by interferon-α. Blood 128 (22):1120

78. Kalmanti L, Saussele S, Lauseker M, Muller MC, Dietz CT, Heinrich L et al (2015) Safety and efficacy of imatinib in CML over a period of 10 years: data from the randomized CML-study IV. Leukemia 29(5):1123–1132

79. Zhang B, Nguyen LXT, Li L, Zhao D, Kumar B, Wu H et al (2018) Bone marrow niche trafficking of miR-126 controls the self-renewal of leukemia stem cells in chronic myelogenous leukemia. Nat Med 24(4):450–462

80. Qiang W, Antelope O, Zabriskie MS, Pomicter AD, Vellore NA, Szankasi P et al (2017) Mechanisms of resistance to the BCR-ABL1 allosteric inhibitor asciminib. Leukemia 31 (12):2844–2847

81. Neviani P, Harb JG, Oaks JJ, Santhanam R, Walker CJ, Ellis JJ et al (2013) PP2A-activating drugs selectively eradicate TKI-resistant chronic myeloid leukemic stem cells. J Clin Investig 123(10):4144–4157

82. Harb JG, Neviani P, Chyla BJ, Ellis JJ, Ferenchak GJ, Oaks JJ et al (2013) Bcl-xL anti-apoptotic network is dispensable for development and maintenance of CML but is required for disease progression where it represents a new therapeutic target. Leukemia 27 (10):1996–2005
83. Agarwal P, Zhang B, Ho Y, Cook A, Li L, Mikhail FM et al (2017) Enhanced targeting of CML stem and progenitor cells by inhibition of porcupine acyltransferase in combination with TKI. Blood 129(8):1008–1020
84. Zhang B, Chu S, Agarwal P, Campbell VL, Hopcroft L, Jorgensen HG et al (2016) Inhibition of interleukin-1 signaling enhances elimination of tyrosine kinase inhibitor-treated CML stem cells. Blood 128(23):2671–2682
85. Agerstam H, Hansen N, von Palffy S, Sanden C, Reckzeh K, Karlsson C et al (2016) IL1RAP antibodies block IL-1-induced expansion of candidate CML stem cells and mediate cell killing in xenograft models. Blood 128(23):2683–2693
86. Jin Y, Yao Y, Chen L, Zhu X, Jin B, Shen Y et al (2016) Depletion of gamma-catenin by histone deacetylase inhibition confers elimination of CML stem cells in combination with imatinib. Theranostics. 6(11):1947–1962
87. Mizoguchi I, Yoshimoto T, Katagiri S, Mizuguchi J, Tauchi T, Kimura Y et al (2013) Sustained upregulation of effector natural killer cells in chronic myeloid leukemia after discontinuation of imatinib. Cancer Sci 104(9):1146–1153
88. Ilander M, Olsson-Stromberg U, Schlums H, Guilhot J, Bruck O, Lahteenmaki H et al (2017) Increased proportion of mature NK cells is associated with successful imatinib discontinuation in chronic myeloid leukemia. Leukemia 31(5):1108–1116
89. Hughes T, Mauro M, Cortes J, Minami H, Rea D, DeAngelo D et al (2019) Asciminib in chronic myeloid leukemia after ABL kinase inhibitor failure. NEJM 381:2315–2326

Current Management and New Developments in the Treatment of Myelodysplastic Syndrome

7

Shukaib Arslan, Samer Khaled, and Ryotaro Nakamura

Contents

7.1   Myelodysplastic Syndrome: Overview

Myelodysplastic syndrome (MDS) refers to a spectrum of heterogeneous hematopoietic stem cell disorders driven by genetic alterations leading to inefficient hematopoiesis, morphologic dysplasia, and peripheral blood cytopenia(s) [1].

S. Arslan · S. Khaled · R. Nakamura (✉)
City of Hope National Medical Center, 1500 E Duarte Rd., Duarte, CA 91010, USA
e-mail: rnakamura@coh.org

S. Khaled
e-mail: skhaled@coh.org

© Springer Nature Switzerland AG 2021
V. Pullarkat and G. Marcucci (eds.), *Biology and Treatment of Leukemia and Bone Marrow Neoplasms*, Cancer Treatment and Research 181,
https://doi.org/10.1007/978-3-030-78311-2_7

Table 7.1 Cytogenetic scoring system. Data from patients in IWG-PM database [2]

Prognostic subgroup; (patients percentage)	Cytogenetic abnormalities	Median survival, years	Median AML evolution, 25%, years
Very good (4%)	−Y, del(11q)	5.4	NR
Good (72%)	Normal, del(5q), del(12p), del(20q), double including del(5q)	4.8	9.4
Intermediate (13%)	del(7q), + 8, + 19, i(17q), any other single or double independent clones	2.7	2.5
Poor (4%)	−7, inv(3)/t(3q)/del(3q), double including − 7/del(7q), complex: 3 abnormalities	1.5	1.7
Very poor (7%)	−7, inv(3)/t(3q)/del(3q), double including −7 del(7q), complex: 3 abnormalities	0.7	0.7

Median age at the time of diagnosis is 70 years [1]. Clinical presentation of MDS ranges from mild asymptomatic cytopenia to severe symptomatic transfusion-dependent cytopenia, recurrent infections, and progression to acute leukemia. Due to its rather variable clinical course, several prognostic models have been developed in the past few decades. The International Prognostic Scoring System (IPSS) was developed by the International MDS Risk Analysis Workshop (IMRAW) based on a combination of cytogenetic, morphologic, and clinical data [2] (Table 7.1).

More recently, Revised International Prognostic Scoring System (IPSS-R) [2] has been developed by the International Working Group for the Prognosis of MDS (IWG-PM) that defines five risk groups (Tables 7.2 and 7.3). These risk stratification strategies have been used to determine the therapeutic intervention, ranging from supportive care to hypomethylating agents (HMA) to allogeneic hematopoietic cell transplantation (HCT). Recently, somatic mutations in several genes (i.e., *TP53, EZH2, ETV6, RUNX1*, and *ASXL1*) were found to hold independent prognostic value in MDS [3]. Thus, a combined analysis of genetic mutations and IPSS-R/IPSS would likely further refine the risk stratification strategy in future.

Table 7.2 IPSS–R scoring values [2]

Prognostic variable	0	0.5	1	1.5	2	3	4
Cytogenetics	Very good	–	Good	–	Intermediate	Poor	Very poor
Bone marrow blasts, %	≤ 2	–	>2– <5%	–	5–10%	>10%	–
Hemoglobin	≥ 10	–	8- <10	<8	–	–	–
Platelet	≥ 100	50– <100	<50	–	–	–	–
Absolute neutrophil count	≥ 0.8	<0.8	–	–	–	–	–

Table 7.3 IPSS–R
categories risk scores

Risk category	Risk score
Very low	≤ 1.5
Low	>1.5–3
Intermediate	>3–4.5
High	>4.5–6
Very high	>6

Diagnostic approach to MDS and associated genetic mutations are discussed in detail in Chap. 1. In addition, patient-related factors such as age, performance status, and comorbidities should be considered in order to determine the best treatment option. Utilizing the risk stratification based on the disease and patient-specific factors, clear goals should be established to care for each patient. For example, for most medically fit patients, the goal would be to achieve long-term survival with the possibility of cure while for less fit patients, the primary goal tends to be to improve patients' quality of life, and/or prolong life.

7.2 CASE 1—High-Risk MDS

A 66-year-old African American male presented with worsening symptoms of fatigue, exertional shortness of breath, generalized weakness, and developed transfusion-dependent macrocytic anemia. His blood count showed hemoglobin of 7 g/dl, MCV 104 fl, WBC count of 6200/µl, and platelet count of 140,000/µl. Review of peripheral blood smear showed dysplastic neutrophils, macrocytosis, and 5% circulating blasts. Bone marrow biopsy displayed trilineage dysplastic features, with excess blasts, (15%) involving hypercellular marrow (70% cellularity). Cytogenetics analysis revealed complex karyotype with monosomy 5, monosomy 7, and 13q deletion. Mutation analysis detected ASXL1, RUNX1, and EZH2 mutations. Patient was started on azacytidine subcutaneous injections daily for 7 days every 4 weeks. He has no significant comorbidities and was referred for allogenic HCT evaluation.

Calculated IPSS-R score for this patient is 8.5 which stratifies him to be in very high-risk group with median survival of 0.8 years and median time to 25% risk of AML progression of 0.73 years.

7.3 Discussion

Hypomethylating agents (HMA, DNA methyltransferase inhibitors)

Azacytidine and decitabine are HMAs, approved by the Food and Drug Administration (FDA) for treatment of MDS. The rationale for hypomethylation therapy was based on the observation that aberrant DNA methylation is a dominant process in patients with MDS. HMAs indirectly deplete methylcytosine, resulting in hypomethylation of promoters of target genes including tumor suppressor genes that are inappropriately methylated, thereby allowing gene expression. Both azacytidine and decitabine are generally well tolerated with proven efficacy and are considered standard first-line therapy for patients with high-risk MDS.

7.3.1 Azacytidine

Azacitidine was synthesized in 1963 and demonstrated activity in four AML trials in the 1970s, resulting in complete remission in 17% to 36% of the patients in these trials [4]. The registration study leading to FDA approval of azacytidine for all MDS subtypes was a phase III trial in which transfusion-dependent MDS patients were randomized to receive azacytidine or supportive care. Patients in the supportive care arm were allowed to cross over to the treatment arm at time of disease progression [5]. Ninety-nine patients were randomized to the treatment arm, in which azacitidine was administered at 75 mg/m^2 daily for 7 days of a 28-day cycle. Of the 92 patients who were randomized to the supportive care arm, 49 patients crossed over to receive active therapy. When these and other CALGB (Cancer and Leukemia Group B) data were analyzed using the International Working Group (IWG) criteria, Silverman et al. reported response rates of 14% complete and partial response (CR and PR) with 30% hematologic improvement [6]. In the treatment arm, there was a significant delay in MDS transformation to AML or death, but not a significant prolongation of survival. Major toxicities included cytopenias, but patients also reported nausea and injection site-related complications.

The efficacy of azacitidine was next explored in a Phase III trial in which higher risk patients with MDS were randomized to receive azacitidine, at the dose used in the registration study, versus conventional care including best supportive care, low-dose cytarabine, or intensive AML-type induction chemotherapy, as selected by investigators prior to randomization [7]. Of the 358 enrolled patients, 179 were randomized to azacitidine and 179 to conventional care, with the majority ($n = 105$) receiving the best supportive care. Overall response rate (ORR) with azacitidine was significantly better than conventional care, 29% versus 21%. With a median follow-up of 21.1 months, median survival was 24.5 months for the azacitidine and 15 months for the conventional care arm (hazard ratio: 0.58, $P = 0.0001$).

The survival benefit for azacitidine was seen in all prognostic subgroups (i.e., poor, intermediate, and favorable cytogenetics) and age groups, including those 75 years old [8].

7.3.2 Decitabine

Decitabine, developed in 1964, was also first explored in AML patients. The Phase III registration trial for MDS randomized 89 patients to receive decitabine, and 81 patients to receive supportive care [9]. Patients received decitabine at a dose of

15 mg/m^2 every 8 h over 3 days, and repeated every 6 weeks. Using IWG criteria, CRs occurred in 9%, PRs in 8%, and hematologic improvement in 13% of patients, for an ORR of 30%. As with azacitidine, the major toxicities of decitabine were hematologic, but unlike azacitidine, there was not a significant delay in transformation to AML or death in this study. Since the two drugs are biologically similar, this difference is often attributed to variation in the patient population enrolled to each study (earlier MDS patients in the decitabine study) and to an inadequate number of cycles of decitabine administration (median of 2). Alternate dosing schedules, including once-daily dosing of decitabine over 5 days in 28-day cycles, were explored in higher risk patients given a median of >5 cycles of therapy, which yielded CR rates equivalent or better than those seen with azacitidine.

A Phase III study in higher risk patients with MDS was conducted in Europe, comparing 119 patients treated with decitabine at the registration study dosing schedule, to 114 patients randomized to best supportive care. While the CR + PR rate was 23% (similar to azacitidine), the study was unable to demonstrate a survival advantage, with patients randomized to drug living a median of 10.1 months and those randomized to the best supportive care living a median of 5.8 months (hazard ratio: 0.88, $P = 0.38$). Progression-free survival (PFS), but not AML-free survival (AML-FS), was significantly prolonged with decitabine compared to the best standard of care (median PFS: 6.6 versus 3.0 months, respectively; HR: 0.68; 95% CI: 0.52–0.88; $P = 0.004$; median AML-FS, 8.8 versus 6.1 months, respectively; HR: 0.85; 95% CI: 0.64–1.12; $P = 0.24$). AML transformation was significantly reduced at 1 year (from 33% with best standard of care to 22% with decitabine, $P = 0.036$) [10].

Recently a single center phase II study of decitabine (20 mg/m^2 for 10 consecutive days) was conducted in 116 patients with transfusion-dependent MDS ($n = 26$), AML (≥ 60 years old; $n = 54$), or relapsed AML ($n = 36$) [11]. In this trial, response rates were higher in patients with TP53 mutation (100% of 21 patients) or unfavorable cytogenetics (67% of 43 patients) than in patients with intermediate or favorable risk cytogenetics (34%) and wild-type TP53 (41%). Maximum clinical response required at least two, and often three or four treatment cycles.

An oral formulation of decitabine combined with the cytidine deaminase inhibitor cedazuridine has similar pharmacokinetics as intravenous decitabine and was approved recently by the FDA for adults with MDS.

7.3.3 Combination Therapy with HMA

Given the low response rates as well as only modest survival impact of HMA therapy alone, there have been attempts to combine additional agents with HMA. A phase II trial of azacytidine (75 mg/m^2/d $\times$ 5 days) in combination with lenalidomide (10 mg/d $\times$ 21 days (28-day cycle) was conducted in patients with higher risk MDS [12]. This study demonstrated the overall response rate (per modified MDS IWG criteria) of 72% (CR: 44%), median CR duration of 17 + months (range: 3–39+), and median OS of 37+ months (range: 7–55+) for CR patients, 13.6 months for the entire cohort (range: 3–55). A three-arm randomized phase II study by The Southwest Oncology Group (SWOG) evaluating azacytidine alone or in combination with lenalidomide or with vorinostat for higher risk myelodysplastic syndromes failed to show clinical advantage of the combination therapy over the control group (azacitidine alone) [12]. Recently, HMA in combination with the Bcl-2 inhibitor venetoclax showed favorable result in AML [13], and this promising combination is being explored in high-risk MDS.

Although these results from HMA trials represent an important advancement in treatment of patients with MDS, 40–50% of patients did not respond to therapy, and most responders experienced disease progression within 2 years of response [14]. In another study, 435 patients with high-risk MDS and formerly classified as refractory anemia with excess blasts in transformation (RAEB-T) were evaluated for outcome after azacitidine failure [15]. The cohort of patients included four different datasets including AZA001, J9950, and J0443 trials and the French compassionate use program. With the median follow-up after azacitidine failure of 15 months, the median OS was 5.6 months, and the 2-year survival probability was 15%. Data on treatment administered after azacitidine failure were available for 270 patients, demonstrating a better outcome associated with allogeneic HCT and investigational agents compared with conventional clinical care.

7.4 Allogeneic HCT

Allogeneic HCT is the only curative therapy available for patients with MDS. However, this treatment is associated with significant risks of transplant-related mortality/morbidity due to engraftment failure, graft-versus-host disease (GVHD), infections, and regimen-related toxicities [16]. As a result, HCT has been generally offered to more fit/younger patients with higher risk disease, and such practice is supported by decision analysis studies in recipients of both myeloablative conditioning (MAC) and reduced intensity conditioning (RIC) HCT [17, 18]. Both patient- and disease-specific factors play integral role in decision-making whether to offer or recommend HCT to a patient with MDS and in predicting transplant outcome [19]. With the recent advances in supportive care, use of RIC regimens, and availability of unrelated and alternative donors (i.e., haploidentical donors), more patients are undergoing HCT now as compared to the past [20–23].

As MDS is generally a slowly progressive disease, and HCT is associated with a significant upfront risk for mortality, the decision-making process for HCT versus no HCT, and optimal timing of HCT remains complex and requires individualized discussions, based on both the patient- and disease-specific criteria.

7.4.1   Who Should Be Considered for Allogeneic HCT?

Patient-Specific Factors: Currently, there is no specific age cut-off for HCT. With advances in supportive care, and use of RIC regimens, even "older" patients can undergo HCT with good outcomes. Studies have shown that older patients between 60 and 70 years of age who have higher risk disease by the IPSS scoring system benefit from HCT with RIC regimen with improved outcome as compared to the patients in same age range who underwent a non-transplant-based therapy [18]. Multiple indices have been developed to predict transplant outcome based on patient comorbidities but the comorbidity index (HCT-CI) developed by Sorror et al. has shown prognostic significance in clinical studies and is being widely used to predict transplant outcome and risk of mortality [20–26].

Disease-Specific Factors: The most important disease-specific factor in MDS is the risk of transformation to acute myeloid leukemia (AML), which would directly affect the survival. Various models have been developed to risk stratify patients with MDS based on disease characteristics predicting survival. These models include the IPSS-, R-IPSS-, and World Health Organization (WHO) classification-based Prognostic Scoring System (WPSS) [2, 24, 25]. Since somatic mutations have shown to predict the risk of progression and response to therapy, an updated scoring system including somatic mutations is being developed.

Patients who have prolonged transfusion-dependent cytopenia refractory to growth factors or HMA are candidates for allogeneic HCT [26]. Percentage of bone marrow myeloblasts is included in the abovementioned scoring systems, but the OS after HCT does not seem to depend on the percentage of myeloblasts in the marrow except in patients with bone marrow myeloblast of less than 5%, where OS seems to be better [27]. Monosomy and complex karyotypes predict poor outcome in MDS secondary to poor response to therapy and increased risk of relapse and reduced survival after HCT. Multiple somatic mutations have been identified in patients with MDS that affect survival, response to therapy, and outcome after HCT [28–32]. Mutations in genes *ASXL1*, *SRSF2*, *RUNX1*, *U2AF1*, and *TP53* are associated with poor prognosis [32]. Combination of *TP53* mutation with complex karyotype is associated with very poor prognosis especially in post-HCT setting [30]. *SF3B1* mutations are associated with favorable prognosis [32]. *IDH 1, IDH 2, TET 2, and DNMT3A* are associated with multilineage dysplasia [32].

Koreth et al. reported the outcome of RIC HCT in elderly patients with MDS, with respect to IPSS and concluded that favored therapy in this patient population varies with the IPSS risk.[18] A total of 514 patients between ages 60 and 70 years with de novo MDS were evaluated. Patients with CMML, isolated 5q- syndrome, unclassifiable MDS, therapy-related MDS and patients who underwent alternate donor HCT were excluded. Outcome of RIC HCT ($n = 132$) stratified by the IPSS risk was compared with best supportive care for patients with non-anemic low/intermediate-1 IPSS ($n = 123$), hematopoietic growth factors for patients with anemic low/intermediate-1 IPSS ($n = 94$), and hypomethylating agents for patients with intermediate-2/high IPSS ($n = 165$). For patients with low/intermediate-1 IPSS MDS, RIC HCT life expectancy was 38 months versus 77 months with non-HCT approaches. For intermediate-2/high

IPSS MDS, RIC HCT life expectancy was 36 months versus 28 months for non-HCT therapies. In conclusion, for low/intermediate-1 IPSS, non-HCT therapy is preferred, whereas for intermediate-2/high IPSS, RIC HCT offers overall and quality-adjusted survival benefit.

Donor Selection: Human leukocyte antigen (HLA) matching serves as the basis of donor identification for allogeneic HCT [33, 34]. Potential donors for allogeneic HCT include matched related/sibling donors (MSD), matched unrelated donor (MUD) from the donor registry, and alternative donors including haploidentical-related donors (haplo), mismatched unrelated donors (MMUD), and cord blood units. Multiple factors that help selecting the best donor include donor's age, gender, degree of HLA match with the recipient [35], ABO blood group, and cytomegalovirus (CMV) serostatus. Algorithms have been developed to select the best donor for HCT [36, 37]. A matched young sibling donor is preferred as first choice. As most patients with MDS are older, and a younger MSD may not be available, a MUD would be preferred [20]. Syngeneic donor HCT has been performed in MDS patients with good outcome [38, 39]. Studies have shown comparable outcomes with MSD and MUD transplants [40].

Timing of HCT: Patients diagnosed with MDS may be recommended to undergo HCT either at the time of diagnosis or at disease progression. Timing of HCT depends on multiple patient and disease factors. Patients who have lower risk disease on R-IPSS at the time of diagnosis and hence lower risk of progression to acute leukemia are usually recommended to undergo HCT at the time of progression. This approach has been shown to offer survival benefit secondary to non-relapse mortality (NRM) associated with earlier HCT [41]. These patients are best managed with supportive care or novel agents developed for this risk group as discussed later in this chapter. There may be high-risk features in some otherwise lower risk patients such as severe transfusion-dependent anemia, severe neutropenia, and high-risk genetics that may encourage the treating physician to consider an earlier HCT. Patients who have higher risk disease at the time of diagnosis are recommended to undergo allogeneic HCT at the time of diagnosis, if otherwise eligible for this intensive therapy [42]. These patients usually undergo therapy with HMA while waiting for donor availability. The timing of transplant is not clear for patients with intermediate-risk disease with some studies showing benefit of an early transplant [41], and some otherwise [17]. Also, somatic mutations are still not a part of the IPSS, and data shows that presence of some mutations may be higher risk in otherwise low- or intermediate-risk disease, different physicians and centers may have different opinions regarding the role of early HCT in this patient population, in the absence of published guidelines.

Role of Pre-HCT Cytoreductive Therapy: Several retrospective studies have shown that the percentage of myeloblasts in the marrow at the time of diagnosis in patients with MDS predicts outcome after allogeneic HCT [43, 44]. Percentage of marrow myeloblasts is hence included in the IPSS [2], and cytoreductive therapy may be used in pre-HCT setting to reduce the marrow blast burden. It is important to note that experts recommend against pre-HCT cytoreductive therapy in high-risk MDS patients with less than 10% marrow blasts [26].

The patient described above (case 1) had multiple high-risk features, including transfusion-dependent anemia, high marrow myeloblast percentage, very high-risk cytogenetics, as well as high-risk somatic mutations. Based on these high-risk features allogeneic HCT was recommended and urgent donor search was initiated. Patient underwent therapy with HMA during the donor search period.

7.5 CASE 2—Low-Risk MDS with Cytopenia

A 75-year-old female presented with fatigue, exertional shortness of breath, generalized weakness, and macrocytic anemia. Her complete blood count showed hemoglobin of 8.5 g/dl, MCV of 108 fl, WBC count of 3500/μL, and platelet count of 176,000/μL. Review of peripheral blood smear showed a few dysplastic neutrophils, macrocytosis, and no circulating blasts. Bone marrow biopsy showed increased cellularity with dysplastic features in erythroid and granulocyte precursors, with no increase in the blast percentage. Cytogenetics analysis showed del (11q), but NGS panel did not identify any mutations. Serum erythropoietin level was at 95. This patient's IPSS-R score is 1 which stratifies her into very low-risk group. Median survival is 8.8 years. She was initiated on treatment with erythropoiesis-stimulating agent (ESA).

7.6 Discussion

Patients with lower risk MDS have low risk of transformation to AML. However, they need to be closely monitored and supportive care is an essential part of the management for these patients. Supportive care involves close monitoring of blood counts, adequate transfusion with blood products, monitoring for iron overload, and use of growth factors when needed.

Transfusion Support: Patients with MDS may present with varying degrees of cytopenia which may be uni- or multilineage. Also, patients may be asymptomatic with milder forms of cytopenia, which could be detected incidentally on routine blood tests. Patients with MDS and asymptomatic mild cytopenia can be closely observed without any therapy with monitoring of blood counts until development of progressive symptomatic disease [1]. Anemia is the most common cytopenia requiring intervention in low-risk MDS. Patients who are transfusion dependent need to have regular monitoring of blood counts and symptom-guided transfusions and other supportive therapies.

Iron overload: Ineffective erythropoiesis requiring frequent red cell transfusions over a period of time can lead to iron overload with a risk of secondary complications particularly in low-risk MDS patients since they enjoy prolonged survival. Ineffective erythropoiesis resulting in increased iron absorption also contributes to iron overload in a subset of these patients who may not be transfusion dependent

[45, 46]. Free iron species can be toxic to organs and can cause liver cirrhosis, endocrinopathies, cardiomyopathy, and bone disorders [46], so it is very important to monitor for iron load and institute therapy in time to prevent complications. There is recent in vitro evidence that iron overload may impair hematopoiesis as well by impairing hematopoietic stem cell function [47]. Persistent dependence on transfusions and elevated ferritin levels have been shown to be associated with reduced survival especially in patients with lower risk MDS [48]. Oral and parenteral iron chelating agents are available for use and clinical trials have shown the feasibility of using deferasirox to lower iron burden in MDS [49, 50]. Retrospective analysis of these trial data has shown improvement in hematopoiesis sometimes multilineage, in a subset of chelated patients [49, 50]. Clinical guidelines recommend using an iron chelating agent in patients with transfusion-dependent MDS for ferritin levels > 1000–2500 ng/ml [45]. The randomized, double-blind, phase II TELESTO trial evaluated the safety and efficacy of deferasirox versus placebo in 225 patients with low or intermediate-1 risk MDS with a transfusion history of 15–75 packed red blood cell units; a serum ferritin of >1000 ng/mL; and normal cardiac, liver, and renal function. Most patients (72.4%) had intermediate-1-risk disease, and mean age of 61 years. Following a 2:1 randomization, patients received either deferasirox 10 to 40 mg/kg per day ($n = 149$) or placebo ($n = 76$).

Participants in the deferasirox group experienced a significantly longer median event-free survival (EFS), compared with the placebo group: 1,440 days versus 1,091 days (HR] = 0.64; 95% CI 0.42–0.96; $p = 0.01$). The 3-year estimated rate of EFS also was greater with deferasirox (61.5 vs. 47.3%), median overall survival, however was not significantly different between the deferasirox and placebo groups (1,907 days vs. 1,509 days; HR = 0.83; 95% CI 0.54–1.28]; $p = 0.2$) [51].

Growth Factor Support: For patient with anemia, the initial treatment is often an erythropoiesis-stimulating agent such as erythropoietin or darbepoetin if serum erythropoietin level is less than 500 units [1, 52]. Low-risk MDS patients, who have erythropoietin levels of less than 100, are most likely to respond to therapy with erythropoietin [1]. About half of these patients who receive growth factor support respond to the treatment with median duration of response of 20–24 months [53].

In patients with MDS who have neutropenia, the absolute neutrophil count responds to myeloid growth factors such as filgrastim (GCSF) but this response does not significantly affect risk of infection and survival [1, 54]. Risk of progression to acute leukemia with the use of myeloid growth factors has been postulated and there is some indication in vitro [55–57] but there has not been a clear clinical evidence. A combination of erythropoietin and GCSF has shown to improve survival in patients with MDS, especially in the patients who require two or less red cell transfusions in 1 month [58]. Similarly, thrombopoiesis-stimulating agents (TPO mimetics) such as eltrombopag or romiplostim have been used in patients who have thrombocytopenia and are platelet transfusion dependent [59–62]. These agents have shown to reduce significant bleeding events, as well as the need for platelet transfusion. It has been shown in clinical studies that the dose of TPO mimetics required to achieve a response in patients with MDS is much higher compared to the dose needed for immune thrombocytopenia [63]. There is, however, concern that TPO mimetics could accelerate progression to AML [64].

Infection prophylaxis: Patients with MDS are at a higher risk of infection compared to their counterparts secondary to neutropenia and impaired neutrophil function. Infections can increase morbidity and mortality in this population [65]. Quinolones are most frequently used as infection prophylaxis in patients with neutropenia [65].

Other therapeutic options: Patients with unchanged transfusion needs on growth factors, or patients who lose response over time to the growth factors should be evaluated for either immune suppressive therapy, HMAs, or other agents that have not been approved for this indication but have been studied. For example, response to therapy with lenalidomide has been evaluated in patients with low-risk MDS who do not have del(5q), and has shown improvement in transfusion requirement in 26% of these patients [66]. The use of immunosuppressive therapy (IST) was analyzed in a large multicenter retrospective study that included 207 patients treated with IST. Red cell transfusion independence was associated with a hypocellular bone marrow (cellularity <20%). Horse ATG plus cyclosporine was more effective than rabbit ATG or ATG without cyclosporine. Other factors such as age, presence of paroxysmal nocturnal hemoglobinuria, or large granular lymphocytosis clones and HLA DR15 positivity did not predict response to IST [67]. A phase II clinical study randomized the low- and intermediate-risk MDS patients to low-dose decitabine versus low-dose azacytidine [68]. There were 81% intermediate-1 risk in this cohort. The overall response rates (ORRs) were 70 and 49% ($P = 0.03$) for patients treated with decitabine and azacitidine, respectively. Rate of transfusion independence was 32 and 16%, respectively ($P = 0.2$). Cytogenetic response rates were 61 and 25% ($P = 0.02$), respectively. With a median follow-up of 20 months, the overall median event-free survival (EFS) was 18 months: 20 and 13 months for patients treated with decitabine and azacitidine, respectively ($P = 0.1$).

7.6.1 Luspatercept

Luspatercept is a fusion protein that blocks transforming growth factor-beta (TGF-b) superfamily signaling by binding to the ligands of the activin II receptor. This altered signaling improves anemia by rescuing late erythroid precursors from apoptosis thereby increasing erythropoiesis in some patients with lower risk MDS. In a phase II study of Luspatercept for the treatment of lower risk MDS, 63% of the patients demonstrated an erythroid response according to the IWG criteria [69]. In a recently reported phase III trial of 229 patients with MDS with ringed sideroblasts (RS) (defined as $\geq 15\%$ RS or $\geq 5\%$ RS with *SF3B1* mutation) and very low, low or intermediate risk by IPSS, who were randomized (luspatercept: $n = 153$, placebo: $n = 76$), transfusion dependence for ≥ 8 weeks was achieved in 38% of the patients in the luspatercept group compared with 13% in the placebo group ($p < 0.001$). Luspatercept was well tolerated with the most common adverse events including fatigue, diarrhea, asthenia, nausea, and dizziness [70]. Luspatercept is now approved for the treatment of anemia in patients with very low- to intermediate-risk MDS-RS patients who have failed an erythropoiesis-stimulating agent and require two more units of red cell transfusion in a period of 8 weeks.

Sotatercept is another novel agent that has shown promising results in improving anemia in patients with lower risk MDS and further studies are ongoing [71].

Treatment goals for patients with low-risk MDS include achieving transfusion independence, improvement in cytopenias, and improved quality of life. The patient described as Case 2 has lower risk MDS and has EPO level <100 and would be a candidate for initial therapy with an ESA.

7.7 CASE 3—Del(5q) Syndrome

A 78-year-old female presented with generalized weakness, mild exertional shortness of breath, and anemia. Her complete blood count showed hemoglobin of 6.5 g/dL, MCV of 99fL, WBC count of 3500/μL, and platelet count of 531,000/μL. Review of peripheral blood smear showed dysplastic neutrophils, macrocytosis, and no circulating blasts. Bone marrow biopsy showed increased cellularity with dysplastic features in erythroid precursors, increased thrombopoiesis with no increase in blast percentage. Cytogenetics showed del(5q). NGS panel showed no mutations. Serum erythropoietin level was at 450.

7.8 Discussion

Some patients with lower risk MDS who have anemia are found to have the cytogenetic abnormality of del(5q32-33), and mildly elevated platelet count, which is commonly referred to as del(5q) syndrome [72, 73]. Identifying this abnormality is important as most of these patients respond very well to therapy with lenalidomide [74–78]. Lenalidomide induces degradation of casein kinase 1A1 which preferentially affects 5q- cells since they are haplo-insufficient for this enzyme by virtue of the chromosomal deletion [79]. Lenalidomide has shown to reduce transfusion need, and ~65–70% of the patients become transfusion independent after lenalidomide treatment [74, 75, 78]. Lenalidomide can induce cytogenetic remission in ~30–40% of these patients [74, 75], and has shown to reduce the risk of transformation to acute leukemia as well as increased survival in patients with lower risk MDS who have del(5q) [80]. It is important to note that patients who have higher risk MDS with del(5q) as part of complex karyotype or have increased marrow blasts, or in association with *TP53* mutation do not respond well to therapy with lenalidomide unlike lower risk patients with del(5q) as the sole cytogenetic abnormality. Most common side effects are fatigue, neutropenia, thrombocytopenia, diarrhea, and pruritus. Neutropenia and thrombocytopenia usually improve with dose adjustment. Although venous thromboembolism was seen, the incidence is much lower than the multiple myeloma population possibly because dexamethasone is not added to the therapy or because lenalidomide is used at much lower doses for patients with MDS.

7.9 Clonal Cytopenia Versus MDS

Somatic mutations are frequently acquired in hematopoietic cells with aging that leads to clonal expansion. Clonal hematopoiesis has shown to be associated with an increased risk of subsequent diagnosis of hematological malignancies and increased mortality, including mortality from cardiovascular disease. Most of these older adults who acquire clonal hematopoiesis during aging do not develop features of MDS like cytopenia and dysplasia and can be considered to have clonal hematopoiesis of indeterminate potential (CHIP). CHIP patients may have one of many stem cell mutations found in MDS without fitting in the diagnostic criteria of MDS. The most common are mutations in *DNMT3A, TET2,* and *ASXL1*. Clonal cytopenia of undetermined significance (CCUS) denotes cytopenia in patients with CHIP who have no features of dysplasia.[81] Differentiation between these different entities characterized by clonal hematopoiesis is shown in Chap. 1, Table 1.4.

7.10 Novel Agents for MDS

Various novel agents are in early stages of clinical development for MDS. Based on early clinical trial data, promising among them include the Bcl-2 inhibitor venetoclax, the anti CD47 antibody magrolimab, the p53 activator APR-246, and the anti-TIM-3 antibody (MBG 453, sabatolimab) [82–85].

References

1. Steensma DP (2018) Myelodysplastic syndromes current treatment algorithm 2018. Blood Cancer J 8(5):47
2. Greenberg PL, Tuechler H, Schanz J, Sanz G, Garcia-Manero G, Sole F et al (2012) Revised international prognostic scoring system for myelodysplastic syndromes. Blood 120(12):2454–2465
3. Lindsley RC, Saber W, Mar BG, Redd R, Wang T, Haagenson MD et al (2017) Prognostic mutations in myelodysplastic syndrome after stem-cell transplantation. N Engl J Med 376 (6):536–547
4. Saiki JH, McCredie KB, Vietti TJ, Hewlett JS, Morrison FS, Costanzi JJ et al (1978) 5-azacytidine in acute leukemia. Cancer 42(5):2111–2114
5. Silverman LR, Demakos EP, Peterson BL, Kornblith AB, Holland JC, Odchimar-Reissig R et al (2002) Randomized controlled trial of azacitidine in patients with the myelodysplastic syndrome: a study of the cancer and leukemia group B. J Clin Oncol: Official J Am Soc Clin Oncol 20(10):2429–2440

6. Silverman LR, McKenzie DR, Peterson BL, Holland JF, Backstrom JT, Beach CL et al (2006) Further analysis of trials with azacitidine in patients with myelodysplastic syndrome: studies 8421, 8921, and 9221 by the Cancer and Leukemia Group B. J Clin Oncol: Official J Am Soc Clin Oncol 24(24):3895–3903

7. Fenaux P, Mufti GJ, Hellstrom-Lindberg E, Santini V, Finelli C, Giagounidis A et al (2009) Efficacy of azacitidine compared with that of conventional care regimens in the treatment of higher-risk myelodysplastic syndromes: a randomised, open-label, phase III study. The Lancet Oncol 10(3):223–232

8. Seymour JF, Fenaux P, Silverman LR, Mufti GJ, Hellstrom-Lindberg E, Santini V et al (2010) Effects of azacitidine compared with conventional care regimens in elderly (>/= 75 years) patients with higher-risk myelodysplastic syndromes. Crit Rev Oncol Hematol 76 (3):218–227

9. Kantarjian H, Issa JP, Rosenfeld CS, Bennett JM, Albitar M, DiPersio J et al (2006) Decitabine improves patient outcomes in myelodysplastic syndromes: results of a phase III randomized study. Cancer 106(8):1794–1803

10. Lubbert M, Suciu S, Hagemeijer A, Ruter B, Platzbecker U, Giagounidis A et al (2016) Decitabine improves progression-free survival in older high-risk MDS patients with multiple autosomal monosomies: results of a subgroup analysis of the randomized phase III study 06011 of the EORTC Leukemia Cooperative Group and German MDS Study Group. Ann Hematol 95(2):191–199

11. Welch JS, Petti AA, Miller CA, Fronick CC, O'Laughlin M, Fulton RS et al (2016) TP53 and decitabine in acute myeloid leukemia and myelodysplastic syndromes. N Engl J Med 375 (21):2023–2036

12. Sekeres MA, Othus M, List AF, Odenike O, Stone RM, Gore SD et al (2017) Randomized phase II study of azacitidine alone or in combination with lenalidomide or with vorinostat in higher-risk myelodysplastic syndromes and chronic myelomonocytic leukemia: North American intergroup study SWOG S1117. J Clin Oncol: Official J Am Soc Clin Oncol 35 (24):2745–2753

13. DiNardo CD, Pratz K, Pullarkat V, Jonas BA, Arellano M, Becker PS et al (2019) Venetoclax combined with decitabine or azacitidine in treatment-naive, elderly patients with acute myeloid leukemia. Blood 133(1):7–17

14. Uy N, Singh A, Gore SD, Prebet T (2017) Hypomethylating agents (HMA) treatment for myelodysplastic syndromes: alternatives in the frontline and relapse settings. Expert Opin Pharmacother 18(12):1213–1224

15. Prebet T, Gore SD, Esterni B, Gardin C, Itzykson R, Thepot S et al (2011) Outcome of high-risk myelodysplastic syndrome after azacitidine treatment failure. J Clin Oncol: Official J Am Soc Clin Oncol 29(24):3322–3327

16. Jurado M, Deeg HJ, Storer B, Anasetti C, Anderson JE, Bryant E et al (2002) Hematopoietic stem cell transplantation for advanced myelodysplastic syndrome after conditioning with busulfan and fractionated total body irradiation is associated with low relapse rate but considerable nonrelapse mortality. Biol Blood Marrow Transplant 8(3):161–169

17. Cutler CS, Lee SJ, Greenberg P, Deeg HJ, Perez WS, Anasetti C et al (2004) A decision analysis of allogeneic bone marrow transplantation for the myelodysplastic syndromes: delayed transplantation for low-risk myelodysplasia is associated with improved outcome. Blood 104(2):579–585

18. Koreth J, Pidala J, Perez WS, Deeg HJ, Garcia-Manero G, Malcovati L et al (2013) Role of reduced-intensity conditioning allogeneic hematopoietic stem-cell transplantation in older patients with de novo myelodysplastic syndromes: an international collaborative decision analysis. J Clin Oncol: Official J Am Soc Clin Oncol 31(21):2662–2670

19. Sorror ML, Sandmaier BM, Storer BE, Maris MB, Baron F, Maloney DG et al (2007) Comorbidity and disease status based risk stratification of outcomes among patients with acute myeloid leukemia or myelodysplasia receiving allogeneic hematopoietic cell transplantation. J Clin Oncol 25(27):4246–4254

20. Kroger N (2013) From nuclear to a global family: more donors for MDS. Blood 122 (11):1848–1850
21. Blaise D, Furst S, Crocchiolo R, El-Cheikh J, Granata A, Harbi S et al (2016) Haploidentical T cell-replete transplantation with post-transplantation cyclophosphamide for patients in or above the sixth decade of age compared with allogeneic hematopoietic stem cell transplantation from an human leukocyte antigen-matched related or unrelated donor. Biol Blood Marrow Transplant 22(1):119–124
22. Blaise D, Nguyen S, Bay JO, Chevallier P, Contentin N, Dhedin N et al (2014) Allogeneic stem cell transplantation from an HLA-haploidentical related donor: SFGM-TC recommendations (Part 1). Pathol Biol (Paris) 62(4):180–184
23. Nguyen S, Blaise D, Bay JO, Chevallier P, Contentin N, Dhedin N et al (2014) Allogeneic stem cell transplantation from an HLA-haploidentical related donor: SFGM-TC recommendations (part 2). Pathol Biol (Paris) 62(4):185–189
24. Greenberg P, Cox C, LeBeau MM, Fenaux P, Morel P, Sanz G et al (1997) International scoring system for evaluating prognosis in myelodysplastic syndromes. Blood 89(6):2079–2088
25. Malcovati L, Porta MG, Pascutto C, Invernizzi R, Boni M, Travaglino E et al (2005) Prognostic factors and life expectancy in myelodysplastic syndromes classified according to WHO criteria: a basis for clinical decision making. J Clin Oncol 23(30):7594–7603
26. de Witte T, Bowen D, Robin M, Malcovati L, Niederwieser D, Yakoub-Agha I et al (2017) Allogeneic hematopoietic stem cell transplantation for MDS and CMML: recommendations from an international expert panel. Blood 129(13):1753–1762
27. Runde V, de Witte T, Arnold R, Gratwohl A, Hermans J, van Biezen A et al (1998) Bone marrow transplantation from HLA-identical siblings as first-line treatment in patients with myelodysplastic syndromes: early transplantation is associated with improved outcome. Chronic Leukemia Working Party of the European Group for Blood and Marrow Transplantation. Bone Marrow Transplant 21(3):255–261
28. Bejar R, Levine R, Ebert BL (2011) Unraveling the molecular pathophysiology of myelodysplastic syndromes. J Clin Oncol 29(5):504–515
29. Bejar R, Stevenson K, Abdel-Wahab O, Galili N, Nilsson B, Garcia-Manero G et al (2011) Clinical effect of point mutations in myelodysplastic syndromes. N Engl J Med 364 (26):2496–2506
30. Bejar R, Stevenson KE, Caughey B, Lindsley RC, Mar BG, Stojanov P et al (2014) Somatic mutations predict poor outcome in patients with myelodysplastic syndrome after hematopoietic stem-cell transplantation. J Clin Oncol 32(25):2691–2698
31. Nikoloski G, Langemeijer SM, Kuiper RP, Knops R, Massop M, Tonnissen ER et al (2010) Somatic mutations of the histone methyltransferase gene EZH2 in myelodysplastic syndromes. Nat Genet 42(8):665–667
32. Malcovati L, Papaemmanuil E, Ambaglio I, Elena C, Galli A, Della Porta MG et al (2014) Driver somatic mutations identify distinct disease entities within myeloid neoplasms with myelodysplasia. Blood 124(9):1513–1521
33. Armitage JO (1994) Bone marrow transplantation. N Engl J Med 330(12):827–838
34. Anasetti C, Amos D, Beatty PG, Appelbaum FR, Bensinger W, Buckner CD et al (1989) Effect of HLA compatibility on engraftment of bone marrow transplants in patients with leukemia or lymphoma. N Engl J Med 320(4):197–204
35. Lee SJ, Klein J, Haagenson M, Baxter-Lowe LA, Confer DL, Eapen M et al (2007) High-resolution donor-recipient HLA matching contributes to the success of unrelated donor marrow transplantation. Blood 110(13):4576–4583
36. Worel N, Buser A, Greinix HT, Hagglund H, Navarro W, Pulsipher MA et al (2015) Suitability criteria for adult related donors: a consensus statement from the worldwide network for blood and marrow transplantation standing committee on donor issues. Biol Blood Marrow Transplant 21(12):2052–2060

37. Dehn J, Spellman S, Hurley CK, Shaw BE, Barker JN, Burns LJ et al (2019) Selection of unrelated donors and cord blood units for hematopoietic cell transplantation: guidelines from the NMDP/CIBMTR. Blood 134(12):924–934

38. Koreth J, Biernacki M, Aldridge J, Kim HT, Alyea EP 3rd, Armand P et al (2011) Syngeneic donor hematopoietic stem cell transplantation is associated with high rates of engraftment syndrome. Biol Blood Marrow Transplant 17(3):421–428

39. Kroger N, Brand R, van Biezen A, Bron D, Blaise D, Hellstrom-Lindberg E et al (2005) Stem cell transplantation from identical twins in patients with myelodysplastic syndromes. Bone Marrow Transplant 35(1):37–43

40. Hows JM, Passweg JR, Tichelli A, Locasciulli A, Szydlo R, Bacigalupo A et al (2006) Comparison of long-term outcomes after allogeneic hematopoietic stem cell transplantation from matched sibling and unrelated donors. Bone Marrow Transplant 38(12):799–805

41. Alessandrino EP, Porta MG, Malcovati L, Jackson CH, Pascutto C, Bacigalupo A et al (2013) Optimal timing of allogeneic hematopoietic stem cell transplantation in patients with myelodysplastic syndrome. Am J Hematol 88(7):581–588

42. Robin M, Porcher R, Ades L, Raffoux E, Michallet M, Francois S et al (2015) HLA-matched allogeneic stem cell transplantation improves outcome of higher risk myelodysplastic syndrome A prospective study on behalf of SFGM-TC and GFM. Leukemia 29(7):1496–1501

43. Guardiola P, Runde V, Bacigalupo A, Ruutu T, Locatelli F, Boogaerts MA et al (2002) Retrospective comparison of bone marrow and granulocyte colony-stimulating factor-mobilized peripheral blood progenitor cells for allogeneic stem cell transplantation using HLA identical sibling donors in myelodysplastic syndromes. Blood 99(12):4370–4378

44. Sierra J, Perez WS, Rozman C, Carreras E, Klein JP, Rizzo JD et al (2002) Bone marrow transplantation from HLA-identical siblings as treatment for myelodysplasia. Blood 100 (6):1997–2004

45. Mitchell M, Gore SD, Zeidan AM (2013) Iron chelation therapy in myelodysplastic syndromes: where do we stand? Expert Rev Hematol 6(4):397–410

46. Angelucci E, Cianciulli P, Finelli C, Mecucci C, Voso MT, Tura S (2017) Unraveling the mechanisms behind iron overload and ineffective hematopoiesis in myelodysplastic syndromes. Leuk Res 62:108–115

47. Tanaka H, Espinoza JL, Fujiwara R, Rai S, Morita Y, Ashida T et al (2019) Excessive reactive iron impairs hematopoiesis by affecting both immature hematopoietic cells and stromal cells. Cells 8(3)

48. Malcovati L (2007) Impact of transfusion dependency and secondary iron overload on the survival of patients with myelodysplastic syndromes. Leuk Res 31(Suppl 3):S2–S6

49. Gattermann N, Finelli C, Porta MD, Fenaux P, Ganser A, Guerci-Bresler A et al (2010) Deferasirox in iron-overloaded patients with transfusion-dependent myelodysplastic syndromes: results from the large 1-year EPIC study. Leuk Res 34(9):1143–1150

50. List AF, Baer MR, Steensma DP, Raza A, Esposito J, Martinez-Lopez N et al (2012) Deferasirox reduces serum ferritin and labile plasma iron in RBC transfusion-dependent patients with myelodysplastic syndrome. J Clin Oncol 30(17):2134–2139

51. Angelucci E, Li J, Greenberg P, Wu D, Hou M, Montano Figueroa EH et al (2020) Iron chelation in transfusion-dependent patients with low- to intermediate-1-risk myelodysplastic syndromes: a randomized trial. Ann Intern Med 172(8):513–522

52. Hellstrom-Lindberg E, Gulbrandsen N, Lindberg G, Ahlgren T, Dahl IM, Dybedal I et al (2003) A validated decision model for treating the anaemia of myelodysplastic syndromes with erythropoietin + granulocyte colony-stimulating factor: significant effects on quality of life. Br J Haematol 120(6):1037–1046

53. Park S, Grabar S, Kelaidi C, Beyne-Rauzy O, Picard F, Bardet V et al (2008) Predictive factors of response and survival in myelodysplastic syndrome treated with erythropoietin and G-CSF: the GFM experience. Blood 111(2):574–582

54. Steensma DP (2011) Hematopoietic growth factors in myelodysplastic syndromes. Semin Oncol 38(5):635–647

55. Kelleher C, Miyauchi J, Wong G, Clark S, Minden MD, McCulloch EA (1987) Synergism between recombinant growth factors, GM-CSF and G-CSF, acting on the blast cells of acute myeloblastic leukemia. Blood 69(5):1498–1503

56. Hoang T, Nara N, Wong G, Clark S, Minden MD, McCulloch EA (1986) Effects of recombinant GM-CSF on the blast cells of acute myeloblastic leukemia. Blood 68(1):313–316

57. Miyauchi J, Kelleher CA, Wong GG, Yang YC, Clark SC, Minkin S et al (1988) The effects of combinations of the recombinant growth factors GM-CSF, G-CSF, IL-3, and CSF-1 on leukemic blast cells in suspension culture. Leukemia 2(6):382–387

58. Jadersten M, Malcovati L, Dybedal I, Della Porta MG, Invernizzi R, Montgomery SM et al (2008) Erythropoietin and granulocyte-colony stimulating factor treatment associated with improved survival in myelodysplastic syndrome. J Clin Oncol 26(21):3607–3613

59. Dickinson M, Cherif H, Fenaux P, Mittelman M, Verma A, Portella MSO et al (2018) Azacitidine with or without eltrombopag for first-line treatment of intermediate- or high-risk MDS with thrombocytopenia. Blood 132(25):2629–2638

60. Mittelman M, Platzbecker U, Afanasyev B, Grosicki S, Wong RSM, Anagnostopoulos A et al (2018) Eltrombopag for advanced myelodysplastic syndromes or acute myeloid leukaemia and severe thrombocytopenia (ASPIRE): a randomised, placebo-controlled, phase 2 trial. Lancet Haematol 5(1):e34–e43

61. Brierley CK, Steensma DP (2015) Thrombopoiesis-stimulating agents and myelodysplastic syndromes. Br J Haematol 169(3):309–323

62. Oliva EN, Alati C, Santini V, Poloni A, Molteni A, Niscola P et al (2017) Eltrombopag versus placebo for low-risk myelodysplastic syndromes with thrombocytopenia (EQoL-MDS): phase 1 results of a single-blind, randomised, controlled, phase 2 superiority trial. Lancet Haematol 4(3):e127–e136

63. Sekeres MA, Kantarjian H, Fenaux P, Becker P, Boruchov A, Guerci-Bresler A et al (2011) Subcutaneous or intravenous administration of romiplostim in thrombocytopenic patients with lower risk myelodysplastic syndromes. Cancer 117(5):992–1000

64. Dodillet H, Kreuzer KA, Monsef I, Skoetz N (2017) Thrombopoietin mimetics for patients with myelodysplastic syndromes. Cochrane Database Syst Rev 9:CD009883

65. Radsak M, Platzbecker U, Schmidt CS, Hofmann WK, Nolte F (2017) Infectious complications in patients with myelodysplastic syndromes: a review of the literature with emphasis on patients treated with 5-azacitidine. Eur J Haematol 99(2):112–118

66. Santini V, Almeida A, Giagounidis A, Gropper S, Jonasova A, Vey N et al (2016) Randomized phase III study of lenalidomide versus placebo in RBC transfusion-dependent patients with lower-risk non-del(5q) myelodysplastic syndromes and ineligible for or refractory to erythropoiesis-stimulating agents. J Clin Oncol 34(25):2988–2996

67. Stahl M, DeVeaux M, de Witte T, Neukirchen J, Sekeres MA, Brunner AM et al (2018) The use of immunosuppressive therapy in MDS: clinical outcomes and their predictors in a large international patient cohort. Blood Adv 2(14):1765–1772

68. Jabbour E, Short NJ, Montalban-Bravo G, Huang X, Bueso-Ramos C, Qiao W et al (2017) Randomized phase 2 study of low-dose decitabine vs low-dose azacitidine in lower-risk MDS and MDS/MPN. Blood 130(13):1514–1522

69. Platzbecker U, Germing U, Gotze KS, Kiewe P, Mayer K, Chromik J et al (2017) Luspatercept for the treatment of anaemia in patients with lower-risk myelodysplastic syndromes (PACE-MDS): a multicentre, open-label phase 2 dose-finding study with long-term extension study. Lancet Oncol 18(10):1338–1347

70. Fenaux P, Platzbecker U, Mufti GJ, Garcia-Manero G, Buckstein R, Santini V et al (2020) Luspatercept in patients with lower-risk myelodysplastic syndromes. N Engl J Med 382 (2):140–151

71. Komrokji R, Garcia-Manero G, Ades L, Prebet T, Steensma DP, Jurcic JG et al (2018) Sotatercept with long-term extension for the treatment of anaemia in patients with lower-risk myelodysplastic syndromes: a phase 2, dose-ranging trial. Lancet Haematol 5(2):e63–e72

72. Jadersten M (2010) Pathophysiology and treatment of the myelodysplastic syndrome with isolated 5q deletion. Haematologica 95(3):348–351
73. Godon C, Talmant P, Garand R, Accart F, Bataille R, Avet-Loiseau H (2000) Deletion of 5q31 is observed in megakaryocytic cells in patients with myelodysplastic syndromes and a del(5q), including the 5q- syndrome. Genes Chromosomes Cancer 29(4):350–352
74. List A, Dewald G, Bennett J, Giagounidis A, Raza A, Feldman E et al (2006) Lenalidomide in the myelodysplastic syndrome with chromosome 5q deletion. N Engl J Med 355(14):1456–1465
75. List A, Kurtin S, Roe DJ, Buresh A, Mahadevan D, Fuchs D et al (2005) Efficacy of lenalidomide in myelodysplastic syndromes. N Engl J Med 352(6):549–557
76. List AF (2008) Lenalidomide in myelodysplastic syndromes. Clin Adv Hematol Oncol 6 (4):271–2, 311
77. List AF, Baker AF, Green S, Bellamy W (2006) Lenalidomide: targeted anemia therapy for myelodysplastic syndromes. Cancer Control 13(Suppl):4–11
78. Fenaux P, Giagounidis A, Selleslag D, Beyne-Rauzy O, Mufti G, Mittelman M et al (2011) A randomized phase 3 study of lenalidomide versus placebo in RBC transfusion-dependent patients with Low-/Intermediate-1-risk myelodysplastic syndromes with del5q. Blood 118 (14):3765–3776
79. Fink EC, Ebert BL (2015) The novel mechanism of lenalidomide activity. Blood 126 (21):2366–2369
80. List AF, Bennett JM, Sekeres MA, Skikne B, Fu T, Shammo JM et al (2015) Extended survival and reduced risk of AML progression in erythroid-responsive lenalidomide-treated patients with lower-risk del(5q) MDS. Leukemia 29(12):2452
81. Steensma DP, Bejar R, Jaiswal S, Lindsley RC, Sekeres MA, Hasserjian RP et al (2015) Clonal hematopoiesis of indeterminate potential and its distinction from myelodysplastic syndromes. Blood 126(1):9–16
82. Garcia JS (2020) Prospects for venetoclax in myelodysplastic syndromes. Hematol Oncol Clin North Am 34(2):441–448
83. Jilg S, Hauch RT, Kauschinger J, Buschhorn L, Odinius TO, Dill V et al (2019) Venetoclax with azacitidine targets refractory MDS but spares healthy hematopoiesis at tailored dose. Exp Hematol Oncol 8(1):9
84. David S, Malki MA, Asch A et al (2020) The first-in-class anti-CD47 antibody magrolimab combined with azacitidine is well-tolerated and effective in MDS patients: phase 1b results. In: Presented at the 2020 European hematology society congress. Abstract S187
85. Borate U, esteve J, Porkka K Knapper S, Vey N, Scholl S et al (2020) Anti TI-3 antibody MBG453 in combination with hyopmrthylating agents in patients with high risk myelodysplastic syndrome and acute myeloid leukemia: a phase 1 study. In: Presented at 25th European hematology association annual meeting 2020 Abstract S185

Chronic Lymphocytic Leukemia (CLL): Biology and Therapy

Tanya Siddiqi

Contents

T. Siddiqi (✉)
City of Hope Medical Center, 1500 E Duarte Rd., Duarte, CA 91010, USA
e-mail: tsiddiqi@coh.org

© Springer Nature Switzerland AG 2021
V. Pullarkat and G. Marcucci (eds.), *Biology and Treatment of Leukemia and Bone Marrow Neoplasms*, Cancer Treatment and Research 181,
https://doi.org/10.1007/978-3-030-78311-2_8

8.1   Introduction and Epidemiology

The World Health Organization (WHO) defines chronic lymphocytic leukemia (CLL) as a low-grade leukemic lymphoproliferative disorder that is distinguishable from small lymphocytic lymphoma (SLL) by its leukemic presentation [1]. The latter is essentially a lymph nodal form of the same disease. CLL/SLL is a disease of malignant clonal B lymphocytes and is the most common hematologic malignancy of the Western world with an incidence of about 5/100,000 persons per year in the United States [2]. Incidence increases with age significantly and the median age at diagnosis is 72 years although about 10% CLL/SLL patients present at age < 55 years. There is a male predominance in an approximately 2:1 ratio. The incidence is higher among Caucasians than other races. About 10% of patients with CLL/SLL report a family history of some lymphoproliferative disorder, so it is suspected that some genetic predisposition occurs in individuals although the exact etiology of CLL/SLL development is largely unknown [3].

8.2   Workup and Diagnosis

Some lymphoproliferative disorders like hairy cell leukemia or the leukemic phases of mantle cell lymphoma, marginal zone lymphoma, or follicular lymphoma, can sometimes masquerade as CLL/SLL and therefore it is critical that correct diagnosis is made given the differences in treatment as well as prognosis. All patients should undergo a history and physical examination (historical review of prior complete blood counts [CBC] may shed some light on how long the patient may have had lymphocytosis for before the actual diagnosis of CLL/SLL) as well as laboratory testing for CBC, peripheral blood smear review, and peripheral blood flow cytometry/immunophenotyping. A bone marrow biopsy is typically not needed to diagnose CLL but should be performed if another lymphoproliferative disorder is strongly suspected as well as for the evaluation of cytopenias, especially prior to starting any therapy. Also, bone marrow biopsy is recommended in patients with persisting cytopenias after treatment in order to uncover disease-related versus therapy-related causes.

   The diagnosis of CLL requires peripheral blood lymphocytosis with the presence of ≥ 5000 monoclonal B-cells/μL for at least 3 months duration. The leukemia cells in peripheral blood are typically small, mature lymphocytes with scant cytoplasm, dense chromatin, and lack prominent nucleoli. Admixed with these mature lymphocytes, there may be some larger or atypical lymphocytes, cleaved lymphocytes, or prolymphocytes. Prolymphocytes in excess of 55% of total lymphocyte count would favor a diagnosis of B-cell prolymphocytic leukemia (B-PLL). Cellular debris called "smudge cells" is often found in the peripheral blood smear of CLL patients.

Presence of monoclonal lymphocytosis but with <5000 B-cells/μL in the peripheral blood and no accompanying lymphadenopathy or organomegaly by physical examination or radiographical imaging, cytopenias, or disease-related symptoms is defined as monoclonal B-lymphocytosis (MBL). The incidence of MBL in the United States is about 3.5% in individuals younger than 40 years and increases with age [4]. In Europe, depending on the sensitivity of the test used, the prevalence ranges from 6.7 to 12% in individuals older than 40 years of age. Progression of MBL to frank CLL can occur at a rate of 1–2% per year. The presence of lymphadenopathy and/or splenomegaly with or without peripheral blood lymphocytosis (if present, must be <5000 B-cells/μL of total lymphocytes) may be pure SLL and should be diagnosed formally with a lymph node biopsy. The presence of any cytopenia caused by bone marrow infiltration by disease is consistent with a diagnosis of CLL regardless of the peripheral blood B-lymphocytosis level or the presence/absence of lymphadenopathy.

8.2.1 Immunophenotyping

Leukemic cells of CLL co-express the T-cell antigen CD5 along with the B-cell surface antigens CD19, CD20, and CD23. These clonal leukemic cells express either surface kappa or lambda immunoglobulin (Ig) light chains with variable intensity. Levels of surface immunoglobulin (Ig), CD20, and CD79b are characteristically of low intensity in CLL cells compared with normal B-cells. In contrast, B-PLL cells do not express CD5 in 50% cases and have brighter CD20 and surface Ig expression. On the other hand, leukemic mantle cell lymphoma cells do not express CD23 even though they do co-express other B-cell surface antigens and CD5.

8.2.2 Additional Testing

If indicated, baseline testing should also include direct antiglobulin (Coombs) test, lactate dehydrogenase (LDH), haptoglobin, reticulocyte count, and bilirubin to evaluate for the presence of associated autoimmune hemolytic anemia. Quantitative immunoglobulin levels should be measured periodically to follow progressive hypogammaglobulinemia and/or any monoclonal gammopathy.

8.3 Prognostic Factors

8.3.1 Cytogenetics/FISH

Interphase FISH assessment of CLL cells can show cytogenetic abnormalities in more than 80% of cases. The most common abnormality is a deletion in the long arm of chromosome 13 (del13q14) ($\sim 55\%$) that harbors the miRNAs miR-15a and

16–1, which may be involved in the pathogenesis of CLL/SLL [5]. In general, isolated del13q is a good prognostic marker characterizing a benign disease course and is often found early in the course of the disease.

Other aberrations include:

- trisomy of chromosome 12 (+12; 10–20%)—prognostic relevance of this is uncertain;
- deletion in the long arm of chromosome 11 (del11q23; 10–25%) harboring the *ATM* gene—these patients typically have bulky lymphadenopathy, rapid disease progression, and reduced overall survival;
- deletion in the long arm of chromosome 6 (del6q); and
- deletion in the short arm of chromosome 17 (del17p13; 5–10%) harboring the tumor suppressor gene *TP53*—del17p is considered the most significant negative prognostic factor in CLL. The TP53 protein normally responds to DNA damage by inducing cell cycle arrest and facilitating DNA repair. It can also induce apoptosis in cells with damaged DNA and in this way, mediates the cytotoxicity of many anticancer agents. Resistance to treatment is a characteristic of *TP53* deletion and has been observed for conventional chemotherapeutic agents including purine analogs (del11q can also confer some resistance to standard chemoimmunotherapy regimens, especially those containing purine analogs). Deletion 17p typically occurs upon relapse after therapy or at the time of disease progression (clonal evolution), although it can be an initial cytogenetic abnormality in ∼5% of patients. A subset of patients may have very poor prognostic *TP53* gene mutations (4–37%) that can be missed on FISH analysis and, therefore, it is advisable to perform next-generation sequencing in addition to FISH before any new treatment is undertaken as there could be therapeutic ramifications of del17p and TP53 mutations. *TP53* mutations are associated with higher genomic complexity in CLL.

8.3.2 IGHV Mutation Status

Somatic hypermutation of the immunoglobulin heavy chain variable region (IGHV) is a normal process in B-cell physiology and is responsible for the diverse immunoglobulin pool. CLL cells that retain this normal process (mutated IGHV) have a better prognosis than CLL cells that lack this genetic feature (unmutated IGHV).

8.3.3 Lymphocyte Doubling Time

A lymphocyte doubling time of < 12 months is associated with a poor prognosis.

8.3.4 Other Prognostic Markers

Next-generation sequencing has led to the identification of novel somatic mutations that can predict the behavior of CLL/SLL in patients [6]. *NOTCH 1* mutations are the most frequent somatic aberrations in CLL, affecting 5–10% newly diagnosed patients, 15–20% of progressing patients in need of frontline therapy, and 30% of Richter transformation patients [7]. *SF3B1* is another recurrently mutated gene in CLL/SLL (5–10% newly diagnosed patients, 15% progressing patients in need of frontline therapy, and 20–25% relapsed and fludarabine-refractory patients). In addition to the poor prognostic effects of mutations in DNA-repair genes (*TP53* and *ATM*), *NOTCH 1*-activating mutations can lead to apoptosis resistance with increased survival of tumor cells. Clinically, *NOTCH* 1-mutated CLL/SLL patients show features associated with poor prognosis and have a high risk of Richter transformation and poor outcome [6, 7]. *NOTCH 1* mutations are associated with unmutated IgVH and trisomy 12, while *SF3B1* mutations are more preferentially associated with del11q and ATM mutations [7]. The precise biological consequence of *SF3B1* mutations in CLL is currently unknown.

ZAP70: This is a T-cell receptor-associated protein tyrosine kinase that is involved in intracellular signaling. Expression of ZAP70 confers a poor prognosis as it is thought to be correlated with unmutated IGHV status in 70% of cases. However, this test has poor reproducibility across different laboratories.

CD38 expression: CD38 is a cyclic ADP ribose hydrolase expressed on the cell surface and is detectable by flow cytometry. Expression of CD38 is also correlated with unmutated IGHV status in 70% of cases and so also confers a poor prognosis.

Beta 2-microglobulin (B2M): levels >3.5 mg/L are associated with a poorer prognosis.

CD49d: CD49d is expressed in ~40% of CLL cases and is a strong independent prognostic marker of survival and treatment need/response in CLL at levels above 30% [8, 9].

Bone marrow biopsy: Typically, >30% of nucleated cells in the bone marrow are CLL/SLL cells. Diffuse pattern of marrow infiltration reflects tumor burden and maybe prognostic but the above-mentioned newer markers have superseded the prognostic value of bone marrow biopsies in general.

8.3.5 Disease Stage

Rai and Binet staging systems are the commonly used staging systems and both divide CLL/SLL patients into low-, intermediate-, and high-risk categories (see Tables 8.1 and 8.2). The CLL International Prognostic Index (CLL IPI) is a predictor of overall survival (OS) and is depicted in Table 8.3.

Prognostic scores range from 0 to 10 and identify 4 risk groups with significantly different rates of OS at 5 years ($p < 0.001$ for all): low-risk patients (score 0–1), 93.2% (95% CI 90.5–96.0); intermediate risk (score 2–3), 79.3% (95% CI 75.5–

Table 8.1 Binet staging system

Binet stage	Clinical features
A	Hemoglobin ≥ 10 g/dL, platelets ≥ 100/L, <3 areas of lymphadenopathy/organomegaly[a]
B	Hemoglobin ≥ 10 g/dL, platelets ≥ 100/L, ≥ 3 areas of lymphadenopathy/organomegaly[a]
C	Hemoglobin <10 g/dL, thrombocytopenia (<100,000/μL), or both

[a]nodal areas: cervical [head and neck], axillary, inguinal (including femoral lymph nodes), spleen, liver

Table 8.2 Rai staging system

Rai stage	Risk category	Clinical features
0	Low	Lymphocytosis alone
1	Intermediate	Lymphadenopathy
2	Intermediate	Hepatosplenomegaly
3	High	Anemia (<11 g/dl)
4	High	Thrombocytopenia (<100,000/μL)

Table 8.3 CLL-international prognostic index

Variable	Adverse factor	Score
Age	>65 years	1
Clinical stage	Binet B/C or Rai I-IV	1
17p13 deletion and/or TP53 mutation	Deleted and/or mutated	4
IGHV mutation status	Unmutated	2
B2M level (mg/L)	>3.5 mg/L	2

83.2); high risk (score 4–6), 63.3% (95% CI 57.9–68.8); very high risk (score 7–10), 23.3% (95% CI 12.5–34.1).

8.4 Case 1: Good Risk CLL, Previously Untreated

A 61-year-old man was noted to have lymphocytosis on routine annual laboratory studies 10 years prior to presentation. White blood cell (WBC) count was 16,000/μL and lymphocytes comprised 60% of all WBC. He was asymptomatic and had no associated anemia or thrombocytopenia. There was no hepatosplenomegaly (HSM) or lymphadenopathy (LAD) on physical examination. Workup with peripheral blood flow cytometry showed B-cell CLL with monoclonal B cells co-expressing CD5, CD19, and CD23. CD20 expression was dim. Cytogenetics and fluorescence in situ hybridization (FISH) showed del13q only. He was maintained on active surveillance over the years. More recently, IGHV testing was performed and found to be mutated. His WBC count now is 23,000/ μL and lymphocytes comprise 75% of all WBC. He is still asymptomatic and remains free of anemia, thrombocytopenia, B symptoms, LAD, and HSM. He continues with observation alone for stage 0 CLL.

8.5 Case 2: Poor Risk CLL, Previously Untreated

A 73-year-old man noted enlarged neck lymphadenopathy, 10-lb weight loss, and night sweats over a period of 6 months. He complained of left upper quadrant discomfort and on physical examination was found to have splenomegaly (palpable 3 cm below left subcostal margin). He underwent a lymph node biopsy of a 2.5-cm left cervical lymph node which revealed small lymphocytic lymphoma (SLL). His laboratory studies at diagnosis showed a white count of 23,000/μL with 75% lymphocytes on the differential count. Peripheral blood flow cytometry confirmed CLL with monoclonal B cells co-expressing CD5, CD19, and CD23. Cytogenetics/FISH at diagnosis showed del11q and IGHV analysis showed unmutated IGHV. Next-generation sequencing was performed and revealed NOTCH- 1 mutation. Hemoglobin at diagnosis was 10.5 g/dL and platelet count was 111,000/μL. Over the next 3 months, his WBC count rose to 55,000/μL and he complained of drenching night sweats 2–3 nights a week. His anemia worsened to 9.5 g/dL with no evidence of immune hemolysis or another etiology for anemia. Platelet count was now lower at 95,000/μL and his neck lymph nodes were also appreciably bigger.

8.6 Indications for Treatment of CLL/SLL

See Table 8.4.

Table 8.4 General indications for initiation of treatment in CLL (IWCLL 2018)

Indication	Description	Precautions
Bone marrow failure	Anemia (e.g., Hb <10 g/dL) and/or thrombocytopenia (e.g., <100,000/μL and dropping)	Require bone marrow study to confirm bone marrow failure
Symptomatic disease	Unintentional weight loss >10% during the past 6 months	Exclude other causative pathologies, e.g., sleep disorder
	Fatigue[a]: ECOG performance status ≥ 2; cannot work or perform usual activities	depression, hypothyroidism, chronic infection/inflammation

(continued)

Table 8.4 (continued)

Indication	Description	Precautions
	Fevers >38 °C for ≥2 weeks without evidence of infection	
	Night sweats for >1 month without evidence of infection	
Splenomegaly	Massive (>6 cm below the left costal margin) or symptomatic (abdominal distention, early satiety, pain) or progressive	
Lymphadenopathy	Massive (>10 cm in longest diameter) or symptomatic or progressive	Exclude infectious lymphadenitis and transformation to diffuse large B-cell lymphoma
Progressive lymphocytosis	Increase in absolute lymphocyte count (ALC) of >50% in 2 months or lymphocyte doubling time (LDT) of <6 months	Baseline ALC for calculation of LDT must be >30 × 10^9/L. LDT needs to be determined by using multiple serial ALC counts (2 weekly ALC for >3 months) to perform linear regression analysis. All other potential causes of changes in ALC (eg, infection, recent use of corticosteroids) need to be excluded. ALC alone should not be used as an indication for treatment
Autoimmune complications	Anemia or thrombocytopenia poorly responsive to corticosteroids	
Extranodal involvement	Symptomatic or functional, e.g., skin, kidney, lung, spine	

[a]Use of fatigue as a sole indication for treatment of patients with CLL requires a careful evaluation and exclusion of all alternative etiologies

8.7 Frontline Treatment Options for CLL/SLL

Before approval of Bruton tyrosine kinase (BTK) inhibitors and venetoclax, most patients with CLL received chemoimmunotherapy as their frontline regimen. The choices included combinations of alkylating agents, nucleoside analogues, and anti CD20 antibodies. Some of the common regimens were FCR (fludarabine, cyclophosphamide, rituximab) for younger patients, BR (bendamustine, rituximab) for fit, older patients, and chlorambucil with rituximab for unfit, older patients. While these regimens may still be appropriate for some younger, low-risk CLL patients, particularly in resource-poor settings, the current strategy is, to avoid the use of conventional chemotherapeutic agents. For Stage 0, asymptomatic patients like the patient described in Case 1 above, the recommendation still is observation alone until there is an indication for therapy.

The use of BTK inhibitors, antiCD20 antibodies, and venetoclax is discussed below.

8.7.1 BTK inhibitors

Ibrutinib

This is a first-in-class, orally bioavailable, selective, potent, small-molecule inhibitor of BTK that covalently binds to its target (cysteine-481 residue near the active site of BTK) thereby interrupting B-cell receptor (BCR) signaling and causing apoptosis of B cells. Early phase studies have shown impressive clinical benefit in CLL/SLL patients with an acceptable safety profile [10–12]. In a Phase Ib-II multicenter trial of 85 patients with relapsed/refractory CLL/SLL, two doses (420 mg or 840 mg daily) of ibrutinib were tested. The overall response rate (ORR) in both groups was 71% with an additional 20 and 15% of patients in each group, respectively, exhibiting partial response (PR) with lymphocytosis (PR-L). Responses were independent of any poor prognostic features including del17p. At 26 months, estimated progression-free survival (PFS) was 75% and OS 83% (median not reached for both). Treatment was well tolerated with predominantly grades 1 and 2 adverse events (AEs), which included (>20% occurrence) diarrhea (usually transient and self-limiting), fatigue, upper respiratory tract infections, cough, arthralgias, rash, pyrexia, and edema. There were 15% grade 3–4 neutropenia events but these did not lead to any treatment discontinuations and were managed with growth factors if needed. Based on the data from the 420-mg cohort of patients (n = 48, ORR 58.3%, no CR), ibrutinib received accelerated US FDA approval in February 2014 in the relapsed/refractory setting. Similarly, in this setting, it was granted approval throughout the European Union in October 2014.

Typically, ibrutinib and the other novel targeted agents can lead to rapid reduction in the size of lymphadenopathy and splenomegaly in CLL/SLL, often in conjunction with a simultaneous increase in peripheral blood lymphocytosis due to redistribution [13]. This phenomenon should not be mistaken for disease progression if all other signs and symptoms of CLL/SLL are improving because it is asymptomatic and transient, although it can take several months to resolve typically. It has led to the revision of iwCLL response criteria in which PR-L has been added as a new response criterion to account for this treatment-related redistribution lymphocytosis.

Ibrutinib can lead to some side effects that one should be aware of as they can affect management decisions: (i) atrial fibrillation—this can occur in up to 10% of patients and should be managed with dose hold and beta-blockers. In most cases, ibrutinib can be restarted safely (often at lower doses) once the atrial fibrillation is optimally managed. (ii) Bleeding risk—concurrent management with warfarin was contraindicated in most clinical trials due to some episodes of major hemorrhage, including life-threatening cerebral hemorrhage, in early trials. The bleeding risk of ibrutinib is due to its interference with BTK-dependent platelet aggregation. Many patients have been treated successfully with ibrutinib in conjunction with low molecular weight heparin products, aspirin, clopidogrel, and novel direct-acting oral anticoagulants, but caution should still be exercised in patients requiring warfarin as the trials excluded these patients due to possible adverse interactions related to fluctuating INR leading to a higher risk of major bleeding. In general, ibrutinib should be held for 3 days before through 3 days after any minor procedure that a patient will undergo, and for 7 days before through 7 days after for any major procedure. (iii) Reactivation of viral hepatitis B and opportunistic infections—this is rare but cases of *Pneumocystis jiroveci* pneumonia as well as aspergillosis among other infections, have been reported. Prophylactic antimicrobial agents are not mandated, but in certain situations like heavily pre-treated patients or combination therapy may warrant these precautions. The low-grade toxicities, such as arthralgias, diarrhea, rash, can be manageable but often affect the quality of life. Certain ibrutinib resistance mutations, like C481S and *PLCG2* mutations, have emerged in CLL, albeit uncommon thus far [14].

Phase 3 Trials of Ibrutinib and CD20 monoclonal antibodies in the Frontline Treatment of CLL

RESONATE 2 [15]: Phase III randomized, open-label, multicenter trial of ibrutinib versus chlorambucil in previously untreated CLL/SLL patients aged 65 years [43]. Among 269 randomized and treated patients, the ORR was 86% in the ibrutinib arm and 35% in the chlorambucil arm ($p < 0.001$) by an independent review. There was a significant improvement in event-free survival (EFS), PFS, and OS with single-agent ibrutinib compared with chlorambucil. Based on these results, ibrutinib was approved by the US FDA for the frontline treatment of patients with CLL/SLL in March 2016; it was also approved in Europe for this setting in May 2016. It is now also being evaluated in combination with various novel targeted agents as well as chemoimmunotherapy to see if further improvements in outcomes can be made in a tolerable fashion.

CLL11 [16]: In the German CLL Study Group CLL11 Phase III trial of 781 previously untreated patients with cumulative illness rating scale (CIRS) > 6 or creatinine clearance 30–69 ml/minute, obinutuzumab + chlorambucil (arm 1) was compared directly with rituximab + chlorambucil (arm 2) and with chlorambucil alone (arm 3). There was a significant improvement in ORR and prolongation of PFS on arm 1 compared with arm 3 as well as on arm 2 compared with arm 3. Median PFS was 26.7 months on arm 1 versus 11.1 months on arm 3 ($p < 0.001$) and 16.3 months on arm 2 versus 11.1 months on arm 3 ($p < 0.001$). Treatment on arm 1 improved OS compared with arm 3 ($p = 0.002$). Treatment on arm 1 improved PFS ($p > 0.001$) and CR rates (20.7% versus 7%) and molecular responses compared with arm 2. Infusion-related reactions were more common on arm 1 compared with arm 2 but there was no difference in the risk of infection.

ALLIANCE [17]: Randomized trial in older CLL patients (65 years and above) treated with ibrutinib or ibrutinib + rituximab or BR in a 1:1:1 fashion. The ibrutinib arms were found to be superior in terms of ORR and PFS than the BR arm.

ECOG E1912 [18]: Randomized trial in 529 CLL patients 70 years or younger comparing ibrutinib + rituximab vs. FCR in a 2:1 ratio. The ibrutinib arm showed longer PFS and OS at a median of 33.6 months of follow-up compared with the FCR arm although these were similar in patients with mutated IGHV specifically.

ILLUMINATE [19]: Randomized trial in 229 CLL patients 65 years or older, or younger patients with comorbidities, of ibrutinib + obinutuzumab vs. chrloambucil + obinutuzumab (1:1). After a median follow-up of 31.3 months, median PFS was significantly longer in the ibrutinib arm (not reached vs. 19 months).

Ongoing trials: Ibrutinib-obinutuzumab ± venetoclax in patients younger than 70 years of age (ECOG-ACRIN) and the same randomization in patients 70 years or older (Alliance).

Acalabrutinib

Second-generation oral, highly selective, BTK inhibitor with potentially fewer side effects than ibrutinib.

ELEVATE-TN is a global, phase 3, multicenter, randomized trial of 535 previously untreated CLL patients who received either acalabrutinib monotherapy or acalabrutinib + obinutuzumab or chlorambucil + obinutuzumab (1:1:1) [20]. At a median follow-up of 28.3 months, the median PFS was significantly longer in both the acalabrutinib arms compared with the chlorambucil arm (not reached vs. 22.6 months) and the grade 3 or higher toxicities were low. Atrial fibrillation rates of any grade were 3–4% in the acalabrutinib arms.

8.7.2 BCL2 inhibitor

Venetoclax

BCL2 is an anti-apoptotic protein that is overexpressed in some B-cell malignancies including CLL. Venetoclax is an oral, BCL2 homology domain 3 (BH3)-mimetic agent that inhibits the antiapoptotic signaling through BCL2 thereby leading to apoptosis of CLL cells.

CLL-14 is an open-label, randomized, phase 3 trial investigating fixed duration treatment with venetoclax for 1 year and obinutuzumab for 6 months compared with chlorambucil + obinutuzumab for 6 months in patients with previously untreated CLL and coexisting comorbidities [21]. 432 patients were randomized 1:1 between the two arms and at a median follow-up of 28.1 months, the PFS was significantly longer in the venetoclax arm and across all risk subgroups. The most common grades 3 and 4 adverse event was neutropenia and about 50% of patients received granulocyte colony-stimulating factor in both arms.

The patient described in Case 2 has poor risk CLL by virtue of having deletion 11q, unmutated IGHV, and NOTCH 1 mutations. These patients have a poor outcome with conventional chemoimmunotherapy and should therefore receive one of the novel agent-containing regimens listed in Table 8.5.

Table 8.5 Recommendations for front-line treatment of CLL in 2021

– Clinical trials
– **No Del17p/TP53 mutation and/or no unmutated IGHV:**
• Ibrutinib/acalabrutinib ± anti-CD20 monoclonal antibody, preferably obinutuzumab
• Venetoclax + obinutuzumab (if 1 year time-limited therapy desired)
• In younger patients (age less than 65 years), FCR can be offered if good risk features of CLL including mutated IGHV, but discuss potential serious side effects with patients carefully
– **Del17p/TP53 mutation and/or unmutated IGHV present:**
• Ibrutinib/acalabrutinib ± anti-CD20 monoclonal antibody
• Venetoclax + obinutuzumab (but consider not stopping venetoclax therapy at 1 year if del17p/TP53 mutation present)

8.8 Case 3: Relapsed/refractory CLL

A 59-year-old woman was diagnosed with CLL/SLL 7 years ago when she was found to have asymptomatic lymphocytosis. The initial WBC count was 37,000/μL with 75% lymphocytes and FISH at diagnosis showed del13q. Within 1 year of diagnosis, her lymphocytes doubled and she developed drenching night sweats, anemia, and thrombocytopenia with hemoglobin of 10 g/dL and, platelet count of 95,000/μL, respectively. She was treated with FCR chemotherapy for six cycles and achieved a complete remission. Two years later she was noted to have new cervical lymphadenopathy as well as lymphocytosis. Peripheral blood FISH now showed del13q and del17p with unmutated IGHV. Over the ensuing few months, she again developed drenching night sweats, rapid lymphocyte doubling time, progressive anemia, and thrombocytopenia. Her laboratory studies showed evidence of autoimmune hemolytic anemia (elevated reticulocyte count, indirect bilirubin, and LDH; low haptoglobin, positive direct antiglobulin test). She was treated with a course of steroids initially and ibrutinib was also initiated. The hemolytic anemia resolved and she had a partial remission initially with ibrutinib but progressed a year and a half later with Richter's transformation.

8.9 Treatment of Relapsed/Refractory Disease

The general management of relapsed/refractory CLL currently involves the sequencing of novel agents. As with frontline therapy, chemoimmunotherapy has largely fallen out of favor in this setting as well. The outcomes with novel agents are inferior in patients who have failed prior chemotherapy as in Case 3 and hence it is important to initiate therapy with these agents upfront in high-risk CLL.

A Phase II trial of ibrutinib in 144 CLL/SLL patients with previously treated del17p CLL (RESONATE-17) showed an ORR of 82.6%, including 17.4% PR-L [22]. The median duration of response and median PFS had not been reached at

13 months follow-up. This study secured ibrutinib's place in the frontline and subsequent management of patients with del17p CLL/SLL.

RESONATE [23]: A Phase III, randomized, controlled, open-label, multicenter trial of 391 patients with relapsed/refractory CLL/SLL in which patients were randomized between ibrutinib and ofatumumab treatment arms. The ORR was significantly higher in the ibrutinib arm compared with ofatumumab (42.6 vs. 4.1%, $p < 0.001$), and PFS ($p < 0.001$), and OS ($p = 0.005$) were significantly improved as well regardless of the presence of poor prognostic indicators. This further confirmed ibrutinib's place in the relapsed setting.

The PI3K inhibitors idelalisib and duvelisib have been FDA-approved for relapsed/refractory CLL but potentially have more serious immune-related side effects of pneumonitis, colitis, and hepatitis than BTK inhibitors and venetoclax and therefore they are not used before these agents typically [24, 25].

MURANO trial [26]: Randomized, open-label, phase 3 trial of 389 relapsed/refractory CLL patients randomly assigned to receive venetoclax for 2 years+ rituximab for 6 months or BR for 6 months. After a median follow-up of 23.8 months, the PFS was significantly higher in the venetoclax arm across all clinical and biologic subgroups. In a recent 5-year update of this study, sustained PFS and OS advantage of the venetoclax arm was reported [27]. Conversion back to minimal residual disease (MRD) detectable testing was confirmed in 47 patients and of these, 19 patients experienced disease progression (PD) subsequently. Unmutated IGHV, del17p, and genomic complexity were associated with higher rates of MRD conversion and subsequent PD after attaining undetectable MRD (uMRD) at the end of 2-year treatment.

Acalabrutinib trials: Phase 1b/2 study of acalabrutinib in 134 relapsed/refractory CLL patients showed an ORR (including PR-L) of 94% across all genomic features [28]. After a median of 41 months, median PFS had not been reached yet. The treatment was well tolerated with the most common side effects being mild-moderate diarrhea (52%) and headache (51%). All grade atrial fibrillation and bleeding events occurred in 7% and 5% of patients, respectively.

In phase 3 ASCEND trial of acalabrutinib monotherapy vs. investigator's choice of idelalisib + rituximab or BR (1:1) in 310 patients, acalabrutinib significantly improved PFS and had an acceptable safety profile [29].

TRANSCEND CLL 004 [30]: This is a Phase 1/2 trial of liso-cel (JCAR017) chimeric antigen receptor (CAR)-T cell therapy in relapsed/refractory patients who have failed at least 2 or 3 lines of therapy including a BTK inhibitor. 23 patients were evaluable in the Phase 1 portion and the majority of these had advanced-stage disease and high-risk features. Median prior lines of therapy were 4 (range 2–11) and almost half the patients had progressed on prior ibrutinib as well as venetoclax. Cytokine release syndrome (CRS) of any grade occurred in 74% of patients, but only 2 patients out of 23 experienced grade 3 CRS and no one had grade 4 or 5 CRS. Neurologic events of any grade were seen in 39% of patients, but only 5 patients experienced grade 3 or 4 neurotoxicity. For the rapid management of these specific toxicities, 74% of patients received tocilizumab and/or dexamethasone.

Overall, the response rate at a median follow-up of 11 months was 81% in the 22 patients evaluable for efficacy (45% CR, 36% PR). In 20 patients with samples evaluable for MRD testing, 65% had uMRD to a level of 10^{-4} (uMRD4) in the bone marrow and 75% had uMRD4 in the peripheral blood. The phase 2 portion of this study is ongoing and provides an excellent option for patients who have progressed on at least two novel targeted therapies in the current era of CLL management.

Allogeneic hematopoietic stem cell transplantation (allo-HSCT) is potentially curative but is only used in a selected minority of patients given its toxicities, older age, and comorbidity of CLL patients. This may still be an option for selected younger high-risk patients, particularly if they have failed chemoimmunotherapy since the response to novel agents appear to be lower in this setting.

Recommendations for treatment of relapsed/refractory CLL in 2020:

- Clinical trials
- Venetoclax + rituximab/obinutuzumab (fixed duration for 2 years)
- Acalabrutinib ± obinutuzumab.

8.10 Complications

8.10.1 *Autoimmune Complications* [31]

A positive antiglobulin (Coombs) test may be observed in up to 30% of patients at some point during the disease course, although it is uncommon (<5%) during early stages. Autoimmune phenomena are relatively frequent, with hemolytic anemia (lifetime risk approximately 10–20%) and thrombocytopenia (lifetime risk approximately 5–10%) occurring most commonly, the combination of which is referred to as Evans syndrome. Autoimmune neutropenia and other autoimmune sequelae are infrequent but more common than in the general population. These autoimmune phenomena occur more commonly with advanced disease or with purine analog treatment and respond to corticosteroids/immunosuppression generally. Rituximab is also a very useful agent. Retreatment with purine analogs is not recommended especially if they caused autoimmune hemolytic anemia as this can recur and sometimes be fatal. Thrombopoietin mimetics (romiplostim, eltrombopag, or avatrombopag) are options for CLL-associated immune thrombocytopenia. If the autoimmune event is resistant to these treatments, more specific CLL-directed therapy is recommended to try and stop the inciting process.

8.10.2 **Infections**

Infections are the most important cause of morbidity and mortality in CLL patients especially infections like sinusitis, pneumonia, and zoster. Immunosuppression due to CLL itself as well as with chemo-, immuno-, and targeted-therapies (especially with agents like fludarabine and alemtuzumab historically and now with ibrutinib) is the cause of recurrent, lingering, or life-threatening viral, bacterial, and fungal infections. We recommend the use of PJP and HSV/VZV prophylaxis routinely. We also recommend the treatment of therapy-induced neutropenia with G-CSF and prophylactic antibiotics. In addition, CLL patients benefit from IVIG infusions, especially when their IgG levels are less than 400 mg/dL. If they experience recurrent/lingering infections, routine use of IVIG every 1–3 months is recommended prophylactically even if their IgG levels are not very low. Vaccinations are also an important mode of prophylaxis, especially against *Streptococcus pneumoniae* and influenza virus. We generally avoid live virus vaccines in patients with CLL. Fungal infections, especially with aspergillus have been described early in course of therapy with ibrutinib.

8.10.3 Richter's Transformation

Transformation to an aggressive large cell B-cell lymphoma from CLL is called Richter's transformation and this can occur in <10% cases, especially in those with poor risk genetic features. Rarely, transformation to Hodgkin lymphoma or another aggressive non-Hodgkin's lymphoma (NHL) like prolymphocytic leukemia or T-cell NHL can occur. Overall, the prognosis is poor with median survival of less than 1 year as responses to treatment are generally short-lived. Features suggestive of transformation include rapid growth of a lymph node group that appears very avid on FDG-PET scan, significant elevation of LDH, and B-symptoms. Aggressive combination chemoimmunotherapy regimens like R-ICE, R-EPOCH, R-CHOP can be tried and if remission is achieved and the patient is a candidate for allo-HSCT with a suitable donor, they should proceed to allo-HSCT which can sometimes lead to long-term remissions. Otherwise, consolidation with CAR-T cell therapy should be considered. For refractory disease, there are ongoing clinical trials currently evaluating the use of PD-L1 antibodies and other checkpoint inhibitors alone and in combination with other agents like ibrutinib. Richter's transformation patients should therefore be considered for clinical trials, especially if standard aggressive chemoimmunotherapy is not effective.

References

1. Jaffe E, Harris N, Stein H, Vardiman J (2001) World Health Organization classification of tumour—pathology and genetics: tumours of haematopoietic and lymphoid tissues. IARC Press, Lyon, France
2. Howlader N, Noone A, Krapcho M, Neyman N, Aminou R, Altekruse S et al (2011) SEER cancer statistics review, 1975–2009. National Cancer Institute, Bethesda, MD

3. Brown JR, Neuberg D, Phillips K, Reynolds H, Silverstein J, Clark JC et al (2008) Prevalence of familial malignancy in a prospectively screened cohort of patients with lymphoproliferative disorders. Br J Haematol 143(3):361–368

4. Strati P, Shanafelt TD (2015) Monoclonal B-cell lymphocytosis and early-stage chronic lymphocytic leukemia: diagnosis, natural history, and risk stratification. Blood 126(4):454–462

5. Hallek M, Cheson BD, Catovsky D, Caligaris-Cappio F, Dighiero G, Döhner H et al (2008) Guidelines for the diagnosis and treatment of chronic lymphocytic leukemia: a report from the international workshop on chronic lymphocytic leukemia updating the national cancer institute-working group 1996 guidelines. Blood 111(12):5446–5456

6. Hallek M (2015) Chronic lymphocytic leukemia: 2015 update on diagnosis, risk stratification, and treatment. Am J Hematol 90(5):446–460

7. López-Guerra M, Xargay-Torrent S, Rosich L, Montraveta A, Roldán J, Matas-Céspedes A et al (2015) The γ-secretase inhibitor PF-03084014 combined with fludarabine antagonizes migration, invasion and angiogenesis in NOTCH1-mutated CLL cells. Leukemia 29(1):96–106

8. Bulian P, Shanafelt TD, Fegan C, Zucchetto A, Cro L, Nückel H et al (2014) CD49d is the strongest flow cytometry-based predictor of overall survival in chronic lymphocytic leukemia. J Clin Oncol 32(9):897–904

9. Tissino E, Pozzo F, Benedetti D, Caldana C, Bittolo T, Rossi FM et al (2020) CD49d promotes disease progression in chronic lymphocytic leukemia: new insights from CD49d bimodal expression. Blood 135(15):1244–1254

10. Advani RH, Buggy JJ, Sharman JP, Smith SM, Boyd TE, Grant B et al (2013) Bruton tyrosine kinase inhibitor ibrutinib (PCI-32765) has significant activity in patients with relapsed/refractory B-cell malignancies. J Clin Oncol 31(1):88–94

11. Byrd JC, Furman RR, Coutre SE, Flinn IW, Burger JA, Blum KA et al (2013) Targeting BTK with ibrutinib in relapsed chronic lymphocytic leukemia. N Engl J Med 369(1):32–42

12. O'Brien S, Furman RR, Coutre SE, Sharman JP, Burger JA, Blum KA et al (2014) Ibrutinib as initial therapy for elderly patients with chronic lymphocytic leukaemia or small lymphocytic lymphoma: an open-label, multicentre, phase 1b/2 trial. Lancet Oncol 15 (1):48–58

13. Woyach JA, Smucker K, Smith LL, Lozanski A, Zhong Y, Ruppert AS et al (2014) Prolonged lymphocytosis during ibrutinib therapy is associated with distinct molecular characteristics and does not indicate a suboptimal response to therapy. Blood 123(12):1810–1817

14. Ahn IE, Underbayev C, Albitar A, Herman SE, Tian X, Maric I et al (2017) Clonal evolution leading to ibrutinib resistance in chronic lymphocytic leukemia. Blood 129(11):1469–1479

15. Burger JA, Tedeschi A, Barr PM, Robak T, Owen C, Ghia P et al (2015) Ibrutinib as initial therapy for patients with chronic lymphocytic leukemia. N Engl J Med 373(25):2425–2437

16. Goede V, Fischer K, Busch R, Engelke A, Eichhorst B, Wendtner CM et al (2014) Obinutuzumab plus chlorambucil in patients with CLL and coexisting conditions. N Engl J Med 370(12):1101–1110

17. Woyach JA, Ruppert AS, Heerema NA, Zhao W, Booth AM, Ding W et al (2018) Ibrutinib regimens versus chemoimmunotherapy in older patients with untreated CLL. N Engl J Med 379(26):2517–2528

18. Shanafelt TD, Wang XV, Kay NE, Hanson CA, O'Brien S, Barrientos J et al (2019) Ibrutinib-rituximab or chemoimmunotherapy for chronic lymphocytic leukemia. N Engl J Med 381(5):432–443

19. Moreno C, Greil R, Demirkan F, Tedeschi A, Anz B, Larratt L et al (2019) Ibrutinib plus obinutuzumab versus chlorambucil plus obinutuzumab in first-line treatment of chronic lymphocytic leukaemia (iLLUMINATE): a multicentre, randomised, open-label, phase 3 trial. Lancet Oncol 20(1):43–56

20. Sharman JP, Egyed M, Jurczak W, Skarbnik A, Pagel JM, Flinn IW et al (2020) Acalabrutinib with or without obinutuzumab versus chlorambucil and obinutuzmab for treatment-naive

chronic lymphocytic leukaemia (ELEVATE TN): a randomised, controlled, phase 3 trial. Lancet 395(10232):1278–1291

21. Fischer K, Al-Sawaf O, Bahlo J, Fink AM, Tandon M, Dixon M et al (2019) Venetoclax and obinutuzumab in patients with CLL and coexisting conditions. N Engl J Med 380(23):2225–2236

22. O'Brien S, Jones JA, Coutre SE, Mato AR, Hillmen P, Tam C et al (2016) Ibrutinib for patients with relapsed or refractory chronic lymphocytic leukaemia with 17p deletion (RESONATE-17): a phase 2, open-label, multicentre study. Lancet Oncol 17(10):1409–1418

23. Byrd JC, Brown JR, O'Brien S, Barrientos JC, Kay NE, Reddy NM et al (2014) Ibrutinib versus ofatumumab in previously treated chronic lymphoid leukemia. N Engl J Med 371(3):213–223

24. Flinn IW, Hillmen P, Montillo M, Nagy Z, Illés Á, Etienne G et al (2018) The phase 3 DUO trial: duvelisib vs ofatumumab in relapsed and refractory CLL/SLL. Blood 132(23):2446–2455

25. Furman RR, Sharman JP, Coutre SE, Cheson BD, Pagel JM, Hillmen P et al (2014) Idelalisib and rituximab in relapsed chronic lymphocytic leukemia. N Engl J Med 370(11):997–1007

26. Seymour JF, Kipps TJ, Eichhorst B, Hillmen P, D'Rozario J, Assouline S et al (2018) Venetoclax-rituximab in relapsed or refractory chronic lymphocytic leukemia. N Engl J Med 378(12):1107–1120

27. Kater AP, Kipps TJ, Eichhorst B, Hillmen P, D'Rozario J, Owen C et al (2020) Five-year analysis of murano study demonstrates enduring undetectable minimal residual disease (uMRD) in a subset of relapsed/refractory chronic lymphocytic leukemia (R/R CLL) patients (Pts) following fixed-duration venetoclax-rituximab (VenR) therapy (Tx). Blood 136:Meeting abstract:125

28. Byrd JC, Wierda WG, Schuh A, Devereux S, Chaves JM, Brown JR et al (2020) Acalabrutinib monotherapy in patients with relapsed/refractory chronic lymphocytic leukemia: updated phase 2 results. Blood 135(15):1204–1213

29. Ghia P, Pluta A, Wach M, Lysak D, Kozak T, Simkovic M et al (2020) ASCEND: phase III, randomized trial of acalabrutinib versus idelalisib plus rituximab or bendamustine plus rituximab in relapsed or refractory chronic lymphocytic leukemia. J Clin Oncol 38(25):2849–2861

30. Siddiqi T, Soumerai JD, Dorritie KA, Stephens DM, Riedell PA, Arnason JE et al (2020) Updated follow-up of patients with relapsed/refractory chronic lymphocytic leukemia/small lymphocytic lymphoma treated with lisocabtagene maraleucel in the phase 1 monotherapy cohort of transcend CLL 004, including high risk and ibrutinib-treated patients. Blood 136:4

31. Fattizzo B, Barcellini W (2019) Autoimmune cytopenias in chronic lymphocytic leukemia: focus on molecular aspects. Front Oncol 9:1435

32. Zain J, Simpson J, Palmer J, Wong J, Dandapani S, Colcher D et al (2018) Phase I study of Yttrium-90 labeled ANTI-CD25 (aTac) monoclonal antibody PLUS BEAM for autologous hematopoietic CELL transplantation (AHCT) in patients with mature T-CELL NON-hodgkin lymphoma, the "a-TAC-BEAM Regimen". Blood 132:296 (Meeting abstract: 611)

Biology and Current Treatment of Myeloproliferative Neoplasms

9

Haris Ali, Vinod Pullarkat, and David Snyder

Contents

9.1 Introduction

William Dameshek first developed the concept of "myeloproliferative disorders" in 1951 to describe a group of bone marrow disorders including chronic myeloid leukemia (CML), polycythemia vera (PV), myelofibrosis (MF), and erythroleukemia [1]. He described them as clonal stem cell disorders in which individual blood cell lineage grew "en masse." CML is the most common among these and is discussed elsewhere in this volume. The current WHO classification of hematological malignancies includes CML, primary myelofibrosis (PMF), essential thrombocythemia (ET), polycythemia vera (PV) chronic neutrophilic leukemia,

H. Ali (✉) · V. Pullarkat · D. Snyder
City of Hope Medical Center, 1500 E Duarte Rd, Duarte, CA 91010, USA
e-mail: harisali@coh.org

D. Snyder
e-mail: dsnyder@coh.org

© Springer Nature Switzerland AG 2021
V. Pullarkat and G. Marcucci (eds.), *Biology and Treatment of Leukemia and Bone Marrow Neoplasms*, Cancer Treatment and Research 181,
https://doi.org/10.1007/978-3-030-78311-2_9

chronic eosinophilic leukemia, and Myeloproliferative neoplasm (MPN), unclas-sifiable under the umbrella of MPN [2]. For the purpose of this chapter, we will focus on the more common entities of PMF, ET, and PV. The phenotype of these entities can overlap to a large degree and they share some common clinical features including hepatosplenomegaly, as well as constitutional symptoms due to aberrant cytokine production, including weight loss, night sweats, fatigue, early satiety, and bone pain. They also share pathophysiological features characterized by elevated peripheral blood counts, hypercellular bone marrow, development of bone marrow fibrosis, and extramedullary hematopoiesis. Over last 2 decades, our understanding of pathophysiology has significantly advanced with the discovery of driver muta-tions. Initially, in 2005, the seminal discovery of a mutation V617F in JAK (Janus kinase)-2 leading to gain of function was described in PV, ET, and PMF [3]. Subsequently, two more driver mutations in *MPL* and *CALR* were discovered [4–6] and one of these three mutations is detected in over 90% of these MPNs. These mutations constitutively activate signaling pathways for hematopoiesis. The basis for the association of the same genotype with different phenotypes among the MPNs remains enigmatic to date.

9.2 Diagnosis

The WHO classification of hematologic malignancies has defined diagnostic criteria for PV, ET, and PMF [2]. A bone marrow biopsy is required at the time of diagnosis which can help differentiate these three types of MPN. *BCR-ABL1* rearrangement has to be excluded as some forms of CML may look similar mor-phologically and phenotypically. Criteria for diagnosis of the individual disorders are listed in Tables 9.1 and 9.2.

9.3 Biology and Genetics of MPN

9.3.1 Driver Mutations

The majority of cases of MPN carry one of three mutually exclusive MPN-restricted mutations (JAK2, MPL, or CALR) that drive myeloproliferation. Each of these three different gene mutations ultimately results in constitutive activation of JAK2-dependent cytokine receptor signaling pathways [7]. CALR and MPL mutations are only found in ET or MF, whereas JAK2 mutation can be present in any of the three MPNs. The distribution of these three mutations among MPN is shown in Fig. 9.1.

A somatic mutation in JAK2 was the first driver mutation discovered in BCR-ABL-negative classical MPN and is the most common [3]. The most common mutation in JAK2 is V617F and results from G to T transition at nucleotide 1849 on

Table 9.1 2016 World Health Organization diagnostic criteria for polycythemia vera and essential thrombocythemia

	Polycythemia vera (PV)[a]	Essential thrombocythemia (ET)[b]
Major criteriav	Hemoglobin >16.5 g/dL (men), hemoglobin >16.0 g/dL (women) or Hematocrit >49% (men) Hematocrit >48% (women) or increased red cell mass (RCM) BM biopsy showing hypercellularity for age with trilineage growth (panmyelosis) including prominent erythroid, granulocytic, and megakaryocytic proliferation with pleomorphic, mature megakaryocytes (differences in size)	Platelet count ≥ 450 X 10^9/L BM biopsy showing proliferation mainly of the megakaryocyte lineage with increased numbers of enlarged, mature megakaryocytes with hyperlobulated nuclei. No significant left-shift of neutrophil granulopoiesis or erythropoiesis and very rarely minor (grade 1) increase in reticulin fibers
	Presence of JAK2 V617F or JAK‹2 exon 12 mutation	Not meeting WHO criteria for BCR-ABL1 + CML, PV, PMF, MDS, or other myeloid neoplasms
		Presence of JAK2, CALR, or MPL mutation
Minor criteria	Subnormal serum erythropoietin level	Presence of a clonal marker (e.g., abnormal karyotype) or absence of evidence for reactive thrombocytosis

[a]PV diagnosis requires meeting either all three major criteria or the first two major criteria and one minor criterion
[b]ET diagnosis requires meeting all four major criteria or first three major criteria and one minor criterion

exon 14 of JAK2 gene on chromosome 9p24.1 resulting in substitution of valine to phenylalanine in the pseudokinase domain. This leads to constitutive ligand-independent activation of JAK2 which is the cognate tyrosine kinase for multiple cytokine receptors including receptors for erythropoietin, thrombopoietin, and granulocyte colony stimulating factor.

The vast majority of PV patients (over 95%) have JAK2 V617F mutation. Among the remainder, about 3% of patients with PV carry JAK2 exon 12 mutations that cause mostly isolated erythrocytosis at the time of diagnosis. JAK2 mutations are present in about ~50% of patients with PV and PMF [8].

Mutations in the thombopoietin receptor gene (*MPL*) mostly occur in exon 10 of the gene located on chromosome 1p34.2. Among these the most common are W515L and W515K occurring in the juxtamembrane domain of the receptor. Other mutations have been described but are less common [6, 8]. MPL mutations are present in about 8% of PMF and 4% of ET patients [8]. Similar to JAK2 mutations, MPL mutations cause constitutive activation of MPL receptor in the absence of TPO and activate downstream signaling [9].

Mutations in calreticulin gene (CALR) were discovered with ET and PMF patients who were JAK2 and MPL mutation negative, occurring in 67% and 88%, respectively [4]. CALR gene is located on chromosome 19p13.13. CALR works

Table 9.2 2016 WHO diagnostic criteria for primary myelofibrosis

	Prefibrotic/Early PMF	Overt PMF
Major criteria	Megakaryocytic proliferation and atypia, without reticulin fibrosis > grade 1c, accompanied by increased age-adjusted BM cellularity, granulocytic proliferation, and often decreased erythropoiesis	Megakaryocyte proliferation and atypia accompanied by either reticulin and/or collagen fibrosis (grade 2 or 3)
	Not meeting WHO criteria for BCR-ABL1 + CML, PV, ET, MDS, or other myeloid neoplasm	Not meeting WHO criteria for BCR-ABL1 + CML, PV, ET, MDS, or other myeloid neoplasm
	Presence of JAK2, CALR, or MPL mutation or in the absence of these mutations, presence of another clonal marker, or absence of minor reactive BM reticulin fibrosis	Presence of JAK2, CALR, or MPL mutation or in the absence, the presence of another clonal marker or absence of evidence for reactive BM fibrosis
Minor criteria	Presence of one or more of the following, confirmed in two consecutive determinations: • Anemia not attributed to a comorbid condition • Leukocytosis ≥ 11 Å $\sim$ 109/L • Palpable splenomegaly • LDH level above the upper limit of the institutional reference range	Presence of one or more of the following confirmed in two consecutives determinations: • Anemia not attributed to a comorbid condition • Leukocytosis ≥ 11 Å $\sim$ 109/L • Palpable splenomegaly • LDH level above the upper limit of the institutional reference range • Leukoerythroblastosis

[a]Diagnosis of prefibrotic/early PMF requires all three major criteria and at least one minor criterion. Diagnosis of overt PMF requires meeting all three major criteria and at least one minor criterion

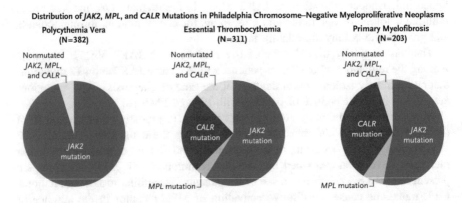

Distribution of *JAK2, MPL,* and *CALR* Mutations in Philadelphia Chromosome–Negative Myeloproliferative Neoplasms

Fig. 9.1 From Klampfl et al N Engl J Med 2013: 369: 2379–90

normally as a chaperone that binds to MPL in endoplasmic reticulum. However, mutant CALR binds to the extracellular domain of MPL receptor and activates signaling. Frameshift mutations in CALR are located on exon 9 and are of two types. Deletions are termed Type 1 (most commonly a 52 base pair deletion) and insertions are classified as Type 2 (most commonly a 5 base pair insertion). Type 1 and Type 2 mutations are equally distributed in ET whereas in PMF Type 1 is more common. They are absent in patients with PV and mutually exclusive with JAK2 and MPL mutations. CALR Type 1 mutation is associated with better survival compared to Type 2 [8].

Only a driver mutation is identified in 50–60% of cases of MPN. In others, in addition to one of the three abovementioned driver mutations, coexisting other mutations may be present at varying frequency. These are not restricted to MPN and may be found in other myeloid neoplasms including acute myeloid leukemia (AML) and myelodysplastic syndrome (MDS) [10, 11]. These include RNA splicing mutations, e.g., SRSF2, SF3B1, U2AF1, and mutations that result in chromatin modifications, e.g., ASXL1, DNMT3A, IDH1/2, EZH2, and TET2, alter signal transduction, e.g., CBL, as well as mutations in the tumor suppressor gene TP53.

There are a some mutations that are considered high risk including ASXL1, IDH1/2, EZH2, SRSF2, and U2AF1, due to shorter overall and leukemia-free survival in MF population [12, 13]. These new discoveries are being utilized in newer prognostic scoring systems to help determine prognosis more accurately. Cytogenetic abnormalities may occur in MPN. Common abnormalities include gains of chromosomes 8 and 9, del 9(p), del 20(q), and del 13(q) among others. Abnormalities like complex karyotype and deletion of 17p are associated with disease progression [2].

A unique feature of MPN is the variability in genotype-phenotype correlation whereby the same driver mutation can be associated with different phenotypes. This is determined by a variety of host factors including age and most importantly patient sex, with PV and ET being more common in women. The incidence of MPN rises with age, being most common after age 60, possibly related to acquisition of mutations that result in clonal hematopoiesis. The precise basis of this variability, however, remains unclear [8].

In most cases, MPN results from sporadic acquisition of somatic driver mutations. In about 7% of cases, there is a familial predisposition to MPN with multiple family members developing the same or another MPN. The genetic basis of such predisposition includes inheritance of single nucleotide variants that predispose to driver mutations, SNPs in TERT gene as well as germline mutations in JAK2 and MPL [8, 14–17].

9.4   CASE 1: Primary Myelofibrosis

A 66-year-old man with no significant prior illness was diagnosed with PMF when he presented in June 2017 with weakness, dyspnea on exertion and night sweats. He was found to have hemoglobin of 6.6 g/dL, WBC count of 3600/μL, and platelet count was 279,000/μL. He became red cell transfusion dependent and required about 1 unit per month. Bone marrow aspirate from June 2018 was hemodilute and showed left-shifted myelopoiesis and trephine biopsy showed a markedly hypocellular marrow with moderate collagen fibrosis and osteosclerosis. There were 1% circulating blasts in peripheral blood but bone marrow did not show increased blasts. Cytogenetics was normal. JAK2 V617F was detected and additionally there were U2AF1 and S34F mutations. Comparison with previous marrow from August 2017 showed increased collagen fibrosis and new U2AF1 mutation suggesting disease progression. Splenomegaly was mild on imaging. He was started on ruxolitinib at 20 mg twice daily with some improvement in constitutional symptoms. He had tried erythropoietin for some time but did not improve anemia. He did not have any history of venous or arterial thrombosis.

He was found to have a histocompatible sibling and underwent allogeneic HCT using fludarabine and melphalan conditioning in January 2019. His HCT course was uneventful and he remains free of disease 1 year and 10 months after HCT.

9.5   Discussion

1. *Initial Diagnosis and prognostication:*

Onset of PMF can be insidious and early stages can be asymptomatic and diagnosed when splenomegaly or elevated WBC count or platelet count is detected on routine clinical examination and laboratory testing. Early prefibrotic phase of PMF may only have leukocytosis or thrombocytosis and bone marrow biopsy is required for differentiation from ET. PMF can cause profound constitutional symptoms and these may be present in up to 50% of cases. In a patient with prior PV or ET progressing to secondary myelofibrosis, features of evolution to myelofibrosis are slowly progressive anemia, leucoerythroblastosis, increasing organomegaly, and constitutional symptoms. Bone marrow biopsy is performed to document transformation and also helps to better prognosticate disease by determining chromosomal abnormalities and percentage of myeloblasts. Often there will be a dry tap and in that case cytogenetics and mutations panel can be done on peripheral blood. There are many prognostic scoring systems used to guide treatment and commonly used ones include Dynamic International Prognostic Scoring System (DIPSS) [18]. Accurate determination of spleen and liver size at diagnosis is important as improvement in size on treatment is a good indication of response which has been used in most of the clinical trials. This patient would be scored "high risk" per

DIPSS criteria (age >65, constitutional symptoms, peripheral blood blasts $\geq 1\%$, and anemia with Hb <10g/dL [5 points]) with a median survival of 1.5 years. By DIPSS Plus which takes into account additional factors like karyotype, transfusion dependency, and platelet count, he would again be classified as "high risk" with a median survival of 16 months [19]. More recently, new prognostic scoring systems have been developed incorporating mutation profile in addition to clinical and pathologic features. MIPSS 70+ v2.0 is one such prognostic scoring system that was devised [20]. Given the fact that he has a high-risk mutation U2AF1 his score would be high risk (8 points) with estimated median survival of 3.5 years. All of these factors as well as the impact of constitutional symptoms and transfusion dependency on his quality of life factored into the decision to proceed to allogeneic HCT.

Both PV and ET can evolve over time to myelofibrosis and this entity is termed secondary myelofibrosis (SMF). Since the prognostic scoring systems discussed above are developed for PMF, a specific prognostic scoring model (MYSEC-PM) has been developed specifically to predict survival in SMF [21].

2. What is the Initial treatment of symptomatic myelofibrosis?

Myelofibrosis can cause profound constitutional symptoms due to elevation of various inflammatory cytokines, i.e., interleukin (IL)-8, IL-2R, IL-12 and IL-15, TNF a, G-CSF, and VEGF [22]. These constitutional symptoms include night sweats, weight loss (>10% of body weight), non-infectious fevers, fatigue, and bone pain all of which severely affects quality of life for patients, in addition to splenomegaly which causes abdominal discomfort and early satiety that contributes to weight loss. A tool called Myelofibrosis Symptoms Assessment Form (MFSAF) has been developed to objectively assess these symptoms and their response to treatment [23]. This assessment is used in various clinical trials that assess treatments for MF. As our patient was symptomatic with constitutional symptoms, treatment with the JAK2 inhibitor ruxolitinib was indicated to relieve these. Ruxolitinib was the first JAK inhibitor approved for the treatment of myelofibrosis based on two randomized phase III trials COMFORT 1 and 2, where it showed significant improvement in splenomegaly and constitutional symptoms. In COMFORT 1 trial, 67% of patients had spleen volume response (defined as reduction in spleen volume of 35% or more on MRI) that was maintained for 48 weeks or more and 46% in ruxolitinib arm had improvement in symptom score by 50% or more at 24 weeks. In COMFORT II that compared ruxolitinib to best available therapy, 29% of patients in ruxolitinib arm achieved spleen volume reduction at 48 weeks [24, 25]. Ruxolitinib is generally well tolerated with anemia and thrombocytopenia being the major side effects and initial dosing of ruxolitinib depends on the platelet count. It is important to mention that approval of ruxolitinib is regardless of patient's JAK2 mutation status. Fedratinib is another JAK inhibitor now approved for intermediate-2 or high-risk primary or secondary MF and its response rate and side effect profile are similar to ruxolitinib except for the side effect of encephalopathy which require monitoring of thiamine level and supplementation if needed [26].

3. *When to perform Allogeneic Hematopoietic Cell Transplant (HCT) for myelofibrosis.*

Allogeneic HCT is currently the only curative option for patient with myelofibrosis either primary or evolving from another MPN. This is offered to patients with advanced symptomatic disease if they are otherwise suitable candidates and have a suitable donor. It may be associated with significant morbidity and mortality related to treatment and thus this decision requires careful consideration and discussion between clinician and patient, particularly with regard to timing of HCT. Various studies have shown it can effectively eliminate malignant clone, resolve marrow fibrosis, and organomegaly over time [27, 28]. It is currently indicated for adverse risk disease patient including intermediate-2 and higher per DIPSS/DIPSS plus, and high risk or higher for patients with MIPSS70+ v2.0 risk disease. Recently, our group published long-term outcome results of a cohort of primary as well as secondary MF patients who underwent reduced intensity allogeneic HCT and showed OS of 65% at 5 years and 59% progression-free survival. Cumulative incidence of relapse at 5 years and non-relapse mortality were only 17% each [27]. These are encouraging results considering the fact that this was a rather high-risk population many of whom having comorbidities that are often observed in MF patients. These results also demonstrate the curative potential of allogeneic HCT for MPN-associated MF.

As our patient in Case 1 remained transfusion dependent on the ruxolitinib treatment and his disease was high risk by DIPSS and DIPSS plus as well as MIPSS70+ v2.0, allogeneic HCT was contemplated due to its curative potential. His brother was identified as a histocompatible donor. Given the propensity of MPNs to be present in multiple members of some families, it is important to evaluate sibling donors carefully for early signs of MPN. He underwent reduced intensity allogeneic HCT using fludarabine and melphalan reduced intensity conditioning regimen. He had no acute and chronic GVHD and remains well almost 2 years after HCT. As expected, there was residual reticulin and collagen fibrosis in his bone marrow biopsy done 3 months after HCT, but JAK2 mutation as well as the previously detected mutations were not detected and donor chimerism was 99%. His peripheral blood counts continue to improve and have almost normalized.

9.6 CASE 2. Polycythemia Vera

A 26-year-old male first developed right lower extremity DVT following a long airplane ride. He subsequently developed a recurrence off anticoagulation 9 months later and at that time was diagnosed with JAK2-mutated PV. His laboratory studies showed hemoglobin of 17g/dL, WBC of 12,000/μ, and platelet count of 545,000/

µL. He had no blasts in the peripheral blood. Patient underwent bone marrow biopsy which showed hypercellular marrow with 80% cellularity, with erythroid, myeloid hyperplasia, and megakaryocytic hyperplasia with myeloblasts <5%. Reticulin stain showed MF-1 fibrosis. Cytogenetics showed 46XY. Molecular studies revealed JAK2 V617F and in addition ASXL1 and EZH2 mutations.

1. *Prognostication and goals of therapy*

Similar to the case with other MPNs, patients with PV have a shortened life expectancy compared to age and sex matched general population [29]. The most common life-threatening complications of PV are thrombosis, both arterial and venous followed by fibrotic progression and leukemic transformation. Initial prognostication and risk assessment are important since that determines the choice of initial treatment and follow-up.

Thrombosis accounted for 41% of deaths in a large prospective study of 1638 patients [30]. At onset of study, 3% of patients had thrombotic history (29% arterial, 14% venous) and after a median follow-up of 2.8 years, 14% of patients in this study had experienced cardiovascular events. In a more recent study of WHO-defined PV patients, thrombosis history was present in 23% at study entry and occurred in 21% (16% arterial, 9% venous) at a median follow-up of 7 years [30, 31].

Based on data from large studies, the two main risk factors for thrombosis are history of prior thrombotic events and age over 60 years. Therefore, patients with either of these risk factors can be considered as having "high-risk" disease, while patients who do not have these two risk factors are at low risk for thrombosis. Other thrombosis risk factors identified include leukocytosis (WBC >15000/µL) and cardiovascular risk factors including hypertension.

Besides thrombosis, leukemic transformation is a major life-threatening complication of PV. Its incidence ranges from 5.5 to 18.7% at 15 years [31]. The presence of cytogenetic abnormalities or certain gene mutations detected on next-generation sequencing including mutations in ASXL1, SRSF2, and IDH2 appears to increase risk of transformation [32, 33]. Eventually almost all patients with PV will evolve into secondary MF. Clues to fibrotic progression include worsening leucoerythroblastosis in peripheral blood, increasing hepatosplenomegaly and peripheral blood cytopenia.

The goals of therapy in PV, therefore, can be broadly summarized as prevention of arterial and venous thrombosis; detection of progression and avoiding leukemic transformation; and providing symptomatic relief from symptoms related to hyperviscosity, splenomegaly, and pruritus, the latter being a dominant symptom in some patients.

2. *Choice of therapy*

The mainstays of initial therapy in PV regardless of risk status are phlebotomy and low-dose aspirin. The goal of phlebotomy is to maintain hematocrit <45% and this is achieved over time by induction of iron deficiency by repeated phlebotomies. This benefit of phlebotomy was established in CYTO-PV study which showed patients with HCT <45% resulted in significantly lower rate of cardiovascular deaths and major thrombotic episodes [34]. The role of low-dose aspirin was established in a large multicenter European study (ECLAP) in which 518 patients were randomized in a double blinded placebo-controlled trial to 100mg of daily aspirin [35]. This study showed that low-dose aspirin significantly lowered risk of thrombotic episodes in these patients.

Cytoreductive therapy is indicated in high-risk patients and hydroxyurea remains the first-line therapy in most patients based on available data from multiple studies [31]. Interferon-alpha including its pegylated form is a first-line option for some patients and unlike hydroxyurea, it can induce molecular responses in a subset of patients. Whether these molecular responses alter the natural history of disease remains unclear and interferon has significantly more toxicity than hydroxyurea. Other options for hydroxyurea-intolerant/refractory patients include oral busulfan and the JAK inhibitor ruxolitinib. Compared to best available therapy, ruxolitinib was more effective in controlling blood counts, reducing spleen size, and providing symptom relief in hydroxyurea-resistant/intolerant PV patients [36]. Its impact on prevention of thrombosis or prolonging leukemia-free survival remains unclear. For patients who experience venous thromboembolism limited data suggest use of systemic anticoagulation in addition to low-dose aspirin. Patients who progress to symptomatic secondary MF should be referred for HCT evaluation if they are suitable candidates given the curative potential of allogeneic HCT.

Our patient in Case 2 can be classified as high-risk PV due to history of thrombosis, and thus he started on treatment to lower cardiovascular risk. He initially started on aspirin, and phlebotomy. His hematocrit normalized after 6 months and he no longer needed phlebotomy. Since he was young and wanted to start a family, he started on treatment of pegylated interferon alpha as it has the possibility of inducing cytogenetic remission and does not have risk of teratogenicity as with hydroxyurea. He tolerated interferon well, although interferon dose had to be adjusted due to development of liver function test abnormalities. His main symptom was aquagenic pruritus. This was controlled with antihistamines, aspirin, and interferon. He also remains on rivaroxaban given the two episodes of venous thrombosis.

9.7 CASE 3: Essential Thrombocythemia

A 45-year-old female presented with mild left upper quadrant abdominal discomfort that prompted a visit to her primary care physician. Laboratory studies showed WBC of 15,500/μL, hemoglobin of 14g/dL, and platelet count of 588,000/μL. No cause of reactive thrombocytosis was evident. She was further evaluated and underwent bone marrow biopsy that showed hypercellular marrow, megakaryocytic hyperplasia, and atypia with MF-1 reticulin fibrosis. Cytogenetics were normal. JAK2 V617F mutation was positive and BCR-ABL1 was negative. Spleen was palpable 6 cm below left costal margin. She denied any constitutional symptoms or erythromelalgia and had no history of thrombotic events.

1. *Initial Diagnosis and Prognostication:*

Our patient in Case 3 was diagnosed with JAK2 mutation-positive ET as her platelet count was >450,000/μL and bone marrow findings of megakaryocyte hyperplasia and atypia in addition to JAK2 mutation met WHO criteria for ET. The major differential diagnosis is prefibrotic phase of PMF (Tables 9.1 and 9.2). Various prognostic models have been developed to predict outcome and guide treatment. Age has a major impact on survival with patients over 70 years of age having a median survival of 8.1 years compared to a median survival of 35 years for patients under 40 years [37]. Recently, a validated prognostic scoring system has been developed (International Prognostic Score for Essential Thrombocytosis, IPSET) that identifies age >60, history of thrombosis, and WBC count over 11,000/ μL as determinants of worse survival [38]. Further refinements have been suggested to this model that incorporates the genetic mutation profile. For example, it is known that patients with CALR-mutated ET have higher platelet counts but less risk of thrombosis compared to ET patients with JAK2 mutations [39] Additional mutations besides the driver mutation can be detected in around 15% of ET patients and some of these including SRSF2, U2AF1, and TP53 may be associated with lower overall survival [37].

A major goal in treatment of ET is prevention of vascular events and thrombotic risk assessment is critical for choice of therapy. Models have also been developed to assess thrombotic risk including IPSET-thrombosis model that takes into account conventional risk factors in addition to JAK2 mutation status [40]. Low-dose aspirin is indicated in most patients unless thrombocytosis is mild and patient is asymptomatic. An algorithm for therapy based on thrombotic risk is shown in Table 9.3. Bleeding, often gastrointestinal, may occur in around 5% of patients with ET and is in some cases associated with acquired von Willebrand disease (due to binding of large vWF multimers by platelets) especially when platelet count is over 1 million.

It is important to note that cytoreductive therapy is indicated in only high-risk patients and should not be used solely for controlling or normalizing platelet count. When such therapy is indicated hydroxyurea is usually the first-line therapy based on a controlled study that showed significantly less thrombotic events in hydroxyurea-treated high-risk patients [41]. Pegylated interferon alfa-2a can be

Table 9.3 Adapted from Tefferi and Pardanani N Engl J Med 2019:381: 2135–44

NCCN and ELN guidelines for risk stratification and treatment in patients with essential thrombocythemia

Guideline	Very low risk1	Low risk1	Intermediate risk1‡	High risk
NCCN[33]				
Patient characteristics	Age ≤ 60 yr, no prior thrombosis, JAK2 V617F mutation absent	Age ≤ 60 yr, no prior thrombosis, JAK2 V617F mutation present	Age >60 yr, no prior thrombosis, JAK2 V617F mutation absent	Age >60 yr, no prior thrombosis, JAK2 V617F mutation present
Rate of thrombosis	0.44%/yr, with no cardiovascular risk factors; 1.05%/yr with risk factors	1.59%/yr with no cardiovascular risk factors; 2.57%/yr with risk factors	1.44%/yr with no cardiovascular risk factors; 1.64%/yr with risk factors	2.36%/yr with no cardiovascular risk factors; 4.17%/yr with risk factors
Management of cardiovascular risk factors	Aspirin, 81–100 mg/day for vascular symptoms§	Aspirin, 81–100 mg/day for vascular symptoms§	Aspirin, 81–100 mg/day for vascular symptoms§	Aspirin, 81–100 mg/day for vascular symptoms§
Treatment	Cytoreductive therapy not recommended as initial treatment	Cytoreductive therapy not recommended as initial treatment	Cytoreductive therapy not recommended as initial treatment	First-line therapy with hydroxyurea or interferon alfa-2a or anagrelide, second-line therapy with hydroxyurea, interferon alfa-2a,‖ or anagrelide, or referral to clinical trial
ELN[18]				
Patient characteristics		Low risk	Intermediate risk	High risk
Rate of thrombosis	–	Score of 0–1, 1.03%/yr	Score of 2, 2.35%/yr	Score ≥ 3, 3.56%/yr
Management of cardiovascular risk factors	–	Low-dose aspirin for microvascular symptoms§	Low-dose aspirin for microvascular symptoms§	Low-dose aspirin for microvascular symptoms§
Treatment				
First line	–	Cytoreductive therapy not recommended for initial treatment	Cytoreductive therapy not recommended for initial treatment	First-line therapy, hydroxy urea or interferon alfa-2a
Second line	–	–	–	Cytoreductive therapy with interferon alfa-2a or anagrelide

used as front-line therapy, particularly for younger patients given its potential to induce molecular response and slow disease progression as in PV, although it is associated with more side effects which make it a less attractive first choice agent. Anagrelide is another approved agent but again its use is limited by its poor adverse event profile, particularly fluid retention and cardiovascular toxicity. In patients who are intolerant or refractory to hydroxyurea, ruxolitinib can be used regardless of JAK2 mutation status [42] but it is important to emphasize that ruxolitinib has not demonstrated disease-modifying potential in MPN.

Erythromelalgia, characterized by erythema, congestion, and burning of distal extremities can be a troubling symptom in some patients. It can precede diagnosis of ET or PV by years. This is usually very responsive to aspirin therapy.

The main goals of treatment in ET are to prevent thrombotic events as well as provide symptom relief. It is important to emphasize that normalization of platelet count is not a goal of therapy. Patients who evolve to post ET MF should be referred for allogeneic HCT if suitable candidates. Our patient in case 3 would be classified as low-risk disease and was therefore treated only with low-dose aspirin (81 mg daily) which she tolerated well.

References

1. Dameshek W (1951) Some speculations on the myeloproliferative syndromes. Blood 6 (4):372–375
2. Arber DA, Orazi A, Hasserjian R et al (2016) The 2016 revision to the World Health Organization classification of myeloid neoplasms and acute leukemia. J Blood 127(20):2391–2405. https://doi.org/10.1182/blood-2016-03-643544
3. Kralovics R, Passamonti F, Buser AS et al (2005) A gain-of-function mutation of JAK2 in myeloproliferative disorders 352(17):1779–1790. https://doi.org/10.1056/NEJMoa051113
4. Klampfl T, Gisslinger H, Harutyunyan AS et al (2013) Somatic mutations of calreticulin in myeloproliferative neoplasms. N Engl J Med 369(25):2379–2390. https://doi.org/10.1056/NEJMoa1311347
5. Nangalia J, Massie CE, Baxter EJ et al (2013) Somatic CALR mutations in myeloproliferative neoplasms with nonmutated JAK2. N Engl J Med 369(25):2391–2405. https://doi.org/10.1056/NEJMoa1312542
6. Pikman Y, Lee BH, Mercher T et al (2006) MPLW515L is a novel somatic activating mutation in myelofibrosis with myeloid metaplasia. PLOS Med 3(7):e270. https://doi.org/10.1371/journal.pmed.0030270
7. Szuber N, Tefferi A (2018) Driver mutations in primary myelofibrosis and their implications. Curr Opin Hematol 25(2):129–135. https://doi.org/10.1097/moh.0000000000000406
8. Spivak JL (2017) Myeloproliferative neoplasms. N Engl J Med 376:2168–2181
9. Defour JP, Chachoua I, Pecquet C, Constantinescu SN (2015) Oncogenic activation of MPL/thrombopoietin receptor by 17 mutations at W515: implications for myeloproliferative neoplasms. Leukemia 30:1214. https://doi.org/10.1038/leu.2015.271
10. Rampal R, Ahn J, Abdel-Wahab O et al (2014) Genomic and functional analysis of leukemic transformation of myeloproliferative neoplasms. Proc Natl Acad Sci 111(50):E5401–E10. https://doi.org/10.1073/pnas.1407792111
11. Stegelmann F, Bullinger L, Griesshammer M et al (2010) High-resolution single-nucleotide polymorphism array-profiling in myeloproliferative neoplasms identifies novel genomic aberrations. Haematologica 95(4):666–669. https://doi.org/10.3324/haematol.2009.013623

12. Guglielmelli P, Lasho TL, Rotunno G et al (2014) The number of prognostically detrimental mutations and prognosis in primary myelofibrosis: an international study of 797 patients. Leukemia 28:1804. https://doi.org/10.1038/leu.2014.76

13. Tefferi A, Finke CM, Lasho TL et al (2018) U2AF1 mutation types in primary myelofibrosis: phenotypic and prognostic distinctions. Leukemia 32(10):2274–2278. https://doi.org/10.1038/s41375-018-0078-0

14. Jones AV, Chase A, Silver RT et al (2009) JAK2 haplotype is a major risk factor for the development of myeloproliferative neoplasms. Nat Genet 41:446–449

15. Hinds DA, Barnholt KE, Mesa RA et al (2016) Germline variants predispose to both JAK2V617F clonal hematopoiesis and myeloproliferative neoplasms. Blood 128:1121–1128

16. Oddsson A, Kristinsson SY, Helgason H et al (2014) The germline sequence variant rs2736100_C in TERT associates with myeloproliferative neoplasms. Leukemia 28:1371–1374

17. Ding J, Komatsu H, Wakita A et al (2004) Familial essential thrombocythemia associated with a dominant positive activating mutation of the c-MPL gene, which encodes for the receptor for thrombopoietin. Blood 103:4198–4200

18. Passamonti F, Cervantes F, Vannucchi AM et al (2010) A dynamic prognostic model to predict survival in primary myelofibrosis: a study by the IWG-MRT (International Working Group for Myeloproliferative Neoplsams Research and Treatment) Blood 115:1703–1708

19. Gangat N, Caramazza D, Vaidya R et al (2011) DIPSS plus: a refined dynamic international prognostic scoring system for primary myelofibrosis that incorporates prognostic information from karyotype, platelet count and transfusion status. J Clin Oncol 29:392–397

20. Tefferi A, Guglielmelli P, Lasho TL et al (2018) MIPSS70+ Version 2.0: mutation and karyotype-enhanced international prognostic scoring system for primary myelofibrosis. J Clin Oncol 36(17):1769–1770. https://doi.org/10.1200/jco.2018.78.9867

21. Passamonti F, Giorgino T, Mora B et al (2017) A clinical-molecular prognostic model to predict survival in patients with post polycythemia vera and post essential thrombocythemia myelofibrosis. Leukemia 31:2726–2731

22. Tefferi A, Vaidya R, Caramazza D, Finke C, Lasho T, Pardanani A (2011) Circulating interleukin (IL)-8, IL-2R, IL-12, and IL-15 levels are independently prognostic in primary myelofibrosis: a comprehensive cytokine profiling study. J Clin Oncol: Official J Am Soc Clin Oncol 29(10):1356–1363. https://doi.org/10.1200/jco.2010.32.9490

23. Mesa RA, Schwager S, Radia D et al (2009) The Myelofibrosis Symptom Assessment Form (MFSAF): an evidence-based brief inventory to measure quality of life and symptomatic response to treatment in myelofibrosis. Leuk Res 33(9):1199–1203. https://doi.org/10.1016/j.leukres.2009.01.035

24. Harrison C, Kiladjian J-J, Al-Ali HK et al (2012) JAK inhibition with ruxolitinib versus best available therapy for myelofibrosis 366(9):787–798. https://doi.org/10.1056/NEJMoa1110556

25. Verstovsek S, Mesa RA, Gotlib J et al (2012) A double-blind, placebo-controlled trial of ruxolitinib for myelofibrosis 366(9):799–807. https://doi.org/10.1056/NEJMoa1110557

26. Talpaz M, Kiladjian J-J (2020) Fedratinib, a newly approved treatmentfor patients with myeloproliferative neoplasm-associated myelofibrosis. Leukemia. https://doi.org/10.1038/s41375-020-0954-2

27. Ali H, Aldoss I, Yang D et al (2019) MIPSS70+ v2.0 predicts long-term survival in myelofibrosis after allogeneic HCT with the Flu/Mel conditioning regimen J Blood Adv 3 (1):83–95. https://doi.org/10.1182/bloodadvances.2018026658

28. Gupta V, Malone AK, Hari PN et al (2014) Reduced-intensity hematopoietic cell transplantation for patients with primary myelofibrosis: a cohort analysis from the center for international blood and marrow transplant research. Biol Blood Marrow Transplant: J Am Soc Blood Marrow Transplant 20(1):89–97. https://doi.org/10.1016/j.bbmt.2013.10.018

29. Hultcrantz M et al (2012) Patterns of survival among patients with myeloproliferative neoplasms diagnosed in Sweden from 1973–2008: a population based study. J Clin Oncol 30:2995–3001

30. Marchioli R, Finazzi G, Landolfi R et al (2005) Vascular and neoplastic risk in a large cohort of patients with polycythemia vera. J Clin Oncol 23(10):2224–2232. https://doi.org/10.1200/jco.2005.07.062
31. Tefferi A, Vannucchi AM, Barbui T (2018) Polycythemia vera treatment algorithm 2018. Blood Cancer J 8:3
32. Tang G et al (2017) Characteristics and clinical significance of cytogenetic abnormalities in polycythemia vera. Haematologica 102:1511–1518
33. Tefferi A et al (2016) Targeted deep sequencing in polycythemia vera and essential thrombocythemia. Blood Adv 1:21–30
34. Marchioli R, Finazzi G, Specchia G et al (2012) Cardiovascular events and intensity of treatment in polycythemia vera. N Engl J Med 368(1):22–33. https://doi.org/10.1056/NEJMoa1208500
35. Landolfi R, Marchioli R, Kutti J et al (2004) Efficacy and safety of low-dose aspirin in polycythemia vera. N Engl J Med 350(2):114–124. https://doi.org/10.1056/NEJMoa035572
36. Vannucchi AM et al (2015) Ruxolitinib versus standard therapy for treatment of polycythemia vera. N Engl J Med 372:426–435
37. Teferri A, Pardanani A (2019) Essential thrombocythemia. N Engl J Med 381:2135–2144
38. Passamonti F, Thiele J, Girodon F et al (2012) A prognostic model to predict survival in 867 World Health Organization-defined essential thrombocythemia at diagnosis: a study by the International Working Group on myelofibrosis research and treatment. Blood 120:1197–1201
39. Rumi E, Pietra D, Ferretti V et al (2014) JAK2 or CALR mutation status defines subtypes of essential thrombocythemia with substantially different clinical course and outcomes. Blood 123:1544–1551
40. Barbui T, Finazzi G, Carobbio A et al (2012) Development and validation of an international prognostic score of thrombpsis in world health organization-essential thrombocythemia (IPSET-thrombosis). Blood 120:5128–5133
41. Cortelazzo S, Finazzi G, Ruggeri M et al (1995) Hydroxyurea for patients with essential thrombocythemia and a high risk of thrombosis. N Engl J Med 332:1132–1136
42. Harrison CN, Mead AJ, Panchal A et al (2017) Ruxolitinib versus best available therapy for ET intolerant or resistant to hydroxycarbamide. Blood 130:1889–1897

Systemic Mastocytosis: Advances in Diagnosis and Current Management

10

Sheeja T. Pullarkat, Winnie Wu, and Vinod Pullarkat

Contents

10.1 Introduction

Mastocytosis is a rare hematologic neoplasm characterized by abnormal proliferation and accumulation of clonal mast cells. Mastocytosis limited to skin is termed cutaneous mastocytosis and will not be discussed further here. Systemic mastocytosis (SM) is characterized by aggregates of atypical mast cells in bone marrow (major criterion for diagnosis defined by World Health Organization) along with

S. T. Pullarkat (✉)
Pathology and Laboratory Medicine, UCLA David Geffen School of Medicine, 10833 Le Conte Avenue, Room AL-134, CHS, Los Angeles, CA, USA
e-mail: SPullarkat@mednet.ucla.edu

W. Wu · V. Pullarkat
Pathology and Laboratory Medicine, Southern California Permanente Medical Group, South Bay Medical Center, 25825 S Vermont Ave, Los Angeles, CA 90710, USA
e-mail: Winnie.Wu@kp.org

V. Pullarkat
e-mail: vpullarkat@coh.org

© Springer Nature Switzerland AG 2021
V. Pullarkat and G. Marcucci (eds.), *Biology and Treatment of Leukemia and Bone Marrow Neoplasms*, Cancer Treatment and Research 181,
https://doi.org/10.1007/978-3-030-78311-2_10

infiltration of other organs among which skin, liver, and spleen are most common. Clinical symptoms arise either from release of mediators from mast cells or in advanced cases from organ dysfunction related to mast cell infiltration. In a large subset of cases, SM coexists with an associated hematological neoplasm (AHN) and in such cases features of the hematologic malignancy dominate the clinical picture. Cases of indolent SM (ISM) comprise the other major subset and are characterized by skin involvement and mediator release symptoms. Rare subsets of SM include aggressive SM (ASM) and mast cell leukemia (MCL) [1].

10.2   Biology and Genetics of SM

KIT is a receptor tyrosine kinase expressed on mast cells and interaction with its ligand, namely, stem cell factor (SCF) supports mast cell differentiation, survival, and proliferation. A gain-of-function point mutation (most commonly *D816V*, though others have been reported) in the tyrosine kinase domain of the *KIT* gene results in ligand-independent activation of the KIT tyrosine kinase [2]. The presence of an activating point mutation at codon 816 of *KIT* is seen in more than 90% of patients and fulfills one of the minor criteria for diagnosis of SM [1]. There is a high correlation between *KIT* mutation detection and the proportion of lesional cells in the samples as well as the sensitivity of the screening method. The question as to whether *KIT* mutation alone is sufficient to cause neoplastic mast cell transformation remains unsettled.

Recent studies have shown that additional mutations identified in SM include *TET2, SRSF2, ASXL1, EZH2, CBL, RUNX1, JAK2,* and *N-RAS* and one or more of these are commonly present in advanced SM which includes SM-AHN, ASM, or MCL and these additional mutations are rare in ISM. The precise prognostic implications of individual mutations are unclear but presence of additional mutations besides *KIT* is associated with worse overall survival [3–5]. In the case of SM-AHN, these additional mutations are acquired at the stem cell level prior to the *KIT D816V* and are present in the mast cell clone as well as the coexisting myeloid malignancy indicating a stepwise pathogenesis [6, 7]. Single cell sequencing studies have shown the *KIT* mutation occurs in early hematopoietic stem cells and is present to a variable extent in different hematopoietic lineages in subtypes of SM [8, 9].

Cytogenetic abnormalities are a feature of SM-AHN. Abnormalities identified are often single chromosomal abnormalities including +8, del(5q), del(7), -7, +13, and del(20q). However, these cytogenetic abnormalities are not unique to SM and are the characteristic of the associated myeloid malignancy [10]. In cases of SM-AHN, the mast cells carry the same cytogenetic abnormality as the AHN again showing their common clonal origin [11]. A specific association exists between SM and t(8;21) AML and coexistence of SM confers an adverse prognosis to this otherwise favorable AML subset [12].

10.3 Diagnosis and Classification of SM

The WHO diagnostic criteria for systemic mastocytosis are listed in Table 10.1. The major criterion for diagnosis is the presence in the bone marrow of multifocal dense aggregates of mast cells (≥ 15 cells in aggregates) with spindled morphology, and cytoplasmic hypogranularity, which is in contrast to normal mast cells which are dispersed, round to oval in shape, with prominent cytoplasmic granularity. These aggregates are often seen in a paratrabecular or perivascular location and are accompanied by many small lymphocytes, histiocytes, fibroblasts, and eosinophils [1]. The paratrabecular lesions are sometimes associated with fibrosis and widening of the bony trabeculae and the perivascular forms are often accompanied by hypertrophy of the associated blood vessels. The associated fibrosis renders the mast cells difficult to aspirate and hence a morphologic evaluation of the bone marrow aspirate will not reflect the extent of underlying mast cell proliferation which requires immunohistochemical evaluation of core biopsy specimens.

The stains that are useful in identifying mast cells in bone marrow include tryptase, which is both sensitive and specific for mast cells. Other immunostains that are useful in identifying mast cells include CD117, CD68, CD43, and CD33. Immunophenotypic aberrancy as manifested by mast cell coexpression of CD25 and, less commonly, CD2 is a minor criterion for diagnosis of SM [1]. CD30 (Ki antigen) has been reported to be preferentially expressed in neoplastic mast cells and earlier studies reported its positivity especially in aggressive SM and MCL. However, further studies have reported CD30 expression in ISM as well. Hence, CD30 while useful as a marker for neoplastic mast cells may not be used as a marker for grading SM [13, 14].

Table 10.1 Diagnostic criteria for SM	*Diagnosis of SM requires major criterion and at least 1 minor criterion or $\geq$ 3 minor criteria*
	Major criterion
	• Multifocal dense infiltrates of mast cells (≥ 15 mast cells in aggregates) detected in bone marrow and/or other extracutaneous organs
	Minor criteria
	• >25% of mast cells in infiltrates are spindle shaped or have atypical morphology or >25% of mast cells in bone marrow aspirates are immature or atypical
	• Detection of activating *KIT* mutation at codon 816 in bone marrow, blood, or an extracutaneous organ
	• Mast cells expressing CD25 with or without CD2 in addition to normal mast cell markers
	• Serum tryptase persistently over 20 ng/mL, unless there is an associated myeloid neoplasm, in which case this parameter is not valid.

The presence of an activating point mutation at codon 816 of *KIT* fulfills one of the minor criteria for diagnosis of SM. Although this mutation occurs at a high frequency in SM, occurring in more than 90% of SM patients, its detection is dependent on sensitivity of assay used and false negative results may occur [15]. Various factors related to testing can lead to negative results on *KIT* mutation assays including low sensitivity of next-generation sequencing assays. Less frequently, other mutations outside of tyrosine kinase domain of *KIT* are present which may be missed in assays directed specifically to *KIT* D816V. In cases where SM is diagnosed, but *KIT* D816 mutation is negative, additional sequencing of the *KIT* gene is recommended since this has therapeutic implications. Since *KIT* mutations can be found in one-third of cutaneous mastocytosis (CM) cases within lesional skin, the WHO criteria for SM specifies that the *KIT* mutation must be identified at an extracutaneous site, most commonly within neoplastic mast cells in the bone marrow.

Should the patient meet the WHO criteria for SM, they can be further subclassified based on a combination of histopathologic and clinical features (Table 10.2). Broadly, the multiple variants fall into two general umbrella categories, with different clinical, prognostic, and therapeutic implications: "advanced systemic mastocytosis" versus "indolent" variants. Encompassed in the "advanced systemic mastocytosis" category are SM-AHN, MCL, and aggressive systemic mastocytosis. The "indolent" variants of SM include smoldering SM and indolent SM.

Majority of patients with advanced SM have SM-AHN. Aside from meeting criteria for SM, SM-AHN demonstrates an associated non-mast cell lineage hematologic neoplasm, which can be diagnosed before, with, or after the diagnosis of SM. The associated hematologic neoplasm can be myeloid or lymphoid/plasmacytic in lineage and can range in aggressiveness from an indolent process to acute leukemia. In 90% of cases, the associated hematologic neoplasm is of myeloid lineage including myelodysplastic syndrome (MDS), myeloproliferative neoplasms (MPN), chronic myelomonocytic leukemia, or acute myeloid leukemia (AML) [1]. Lymphoid neoplasms associated with SM are not clonally related to the

Table 10.2 Variants of SM	*All variants should meet general criteria for SM*
	Indolent variants (skin lesions almost invariably present)
	• Indolent SM (low mast cell burden, No C findings, no hematologic neoplasm)
	• Smoldering SM (B findings, high mast cell burden, no hematologic neoplasm)
	Advanced variants (skin lesions uncommon)
	• SM-AHN
	• Aggressive SM (C findings present)
	• Mast cell leukemia ($\geq 20\%$ mast cells in bone marrow aspirate smears)

coexisting SM [16]. A subset of AML with the (8;21) *RUNX1-RUNX1T1* translocation may show concurrent SM, and the associated mast cell infiltrate may be masked by the acute leukemia infiltrate at initial diagnosis and may not become apparent until following treatment [17]. It is critical to examine bone marrow core biopsy (not aspirate) specimens by immunohistochemistry for mast cell infiltrate if D816 or another activating *KIT* mutation is detected in myeloid malignancies associated with SM since coexisting SM has adverse prognostic impact especially in AML. Skin involvement as well as symptoms related to mast cell mediator release do not seem to occur in SM-AHN. In most cases, the disease course and prognosis are primarily determined by the associated hematologic neoplasm. Therefore, it is important that the associated hematologic neoplasm is separately designated and classified according to defined WHO criteria.

Mast cell leukemia is an aggressive variant of SM. It is highly lethal with an overall survival of <1 year. On pathology, it is characterized by the presence of immature mast cells, which are round rather than spindled, and range in levels of immaturity from bilobated/multilobated promastocytes to metachromatically granulated blasts to scantly granular but tryptase-positive blasts. These immature mast cells diffusely infiltrate the bone marrow. By definition, the neoplastic mast cells should comprise ≥ 20% of cells on aspirate smears [1]. Though it represents the leukemic variant of SM, it is more common for MCL to demonstrate <10% circulating mast cells. Typically, evidence of organ dysfunction secondary to malignant mast cell infiltration is apparent at presentation.

The remaining subtypes of SM are stratified according to clinical aggressiveness and extent of mast cell infiltrate. Provided that MCL and SM-AHN are excluded, if there is evidence of organ dysfunction (defined as the "C findings" in Table 10.3), the diagnosis would be ASM [3]. Aggressive SM most commonly shows organ damage in the form of hematologic or liver dysfunction. Gastrointestinal symptoms (malabsorption and weight loss) count as an organ dysfunction only if biopsies document gastrointestinal mast cell infiltrates as cause of the symptoms. In ASM, the bone marrow aspirate smear (not biopsy) mast cells comprise ≤ 5% of marrow cellularity. Cases in which marrow aspirate mast cells are >5% but <20% are diagnosed as aggressive SM in transformation (to MCL), whereas cases with marrow aspirate mast cells ≥ 20% represent frank MCL [1].

Absence of organ dysfunction characterizes smoldering SM, indolent SM, and the very rare entity termed bone marrow mastocytosis. They differ mainly in the extent of mast cell burden in the marrow, spleen, and liver, with a higher burden of disease in smoldering systemic mastocytosis, defined as the presence of two or more "B findings" (Table 10.3). Indolent SM and bone marrow mastocytosis both show low burden of disease, and they differ only in the presence or absence of skin lesions, respectively [1]. Smoldering SM often remains stable for many years, though progression to aggressive SM or MCL can occur.

Table 10.3 B (disease burden) and C (cytoreduction requiring) findings of SM

B findings
• High mast cell burden ($\geq$ 30% mast cells on bone marrow biopsy, tryptase $\geq$ 200 ng/ml)
• Slight blood count abnormalities with no definite AHN
• Hepatosplenomegaly without functional impairment or lymphadenopathy
C findings
• Bone marrow dysfunction from mast cell infiltration (absolute neutrophil count <1000/ μL, hemoglobin <10 g/dL, and platelet count <100,000/μL)
• Hepatic dysfunction with or without portal hypertension
• Hypersplenism
• Bone lesions (except osteoporosis)
• Malabsorption syndrome from mast cell infiltration of gut

10.3.1   Case 1. SM-AHN

A 37-year-old male presented with pruritus without a rash and then developed pancytopenia (WBC 4100μL, hemoglobin 10.1 g/dL, platelet count 25,000/μL) for which he underwent a bone marrow biopsy. Bone marrow had 100% cellularity and revealed increase of blasts of 5–10%. In addition, the bone marrow biopsy showed clusters of atypical spindle-shaped mast cells with aberrant expression of CD25 as well as *KIT* D816V mutation. Tryptase level was 3.1 μg/L. Megakaryocytes were increased in number and showed dysplastic morphology. There was moderate reticulin fibrosis (MF 2 of 3). Next-generation sequencing (NGS) revealed mutations in *RUNX1*, *U2AF1*, and *CBL* in addition to *KIT*. Cytogenetics revealed trisomy 8. He underwent a haploidentical stem cell transplant from his brother after fludarabine and total body irradiation (1200 cGy) conditioning followed by GVHD prophylaxis with cyclophosphamide, tacrolimus, and mycophenolate mofetil. His bone marrow biopsy on day 34 after transplantation showed persistent mast cell infiltrate (5% of cellularity) but no increased blasts, normal cytogenetics, and absence of previously detected mutations by NGS. Chimerism studies showed 99.14% donor DNA. He continues to remain in remission 2 years after his transplant and is off all immunosuppression with no evidence of graft versus host disease.

Based on the clinicopathologic and molecular findings, Case 1 can be classified as SM-AHN; in this case, the AHN being MDS with excess blasts-1 which dominated the clinical picture as is typical with most cases of SM-AHN. Although he had symptoms of itching, skin lesions of SM were absent as is typically the case with SM-AHN. The presence of additional mutations besides *KIT* D816V as well as cytogenetic abnormality is also typical of SM-AHN. The treatment would primarily be that of MDS which would address the associated SM since the two entities are clonally the same. Therefore, the decision was made to proceed to allo-HSCT, given his age as well as excellent performance status and lack or organ dysfunction from the associated SM. Due to the lack of matched sibling or unrelated donor, a decision was made to perform haploidentical HSCT from his brother and patient had an excellent outcome. Although there was a persistent bone marrow infiltrate of neoplastic mast cells at day 34 after HSCT, this is often seen in the case of SM-AHN after HSCT and does not require any intervention as long as there is no evidence of the original AHN.

10.3.2   Case 2. ISM

A 61-year-old male developed a pruritic rash of small erythematous to brown papules on his posterior thigh that spread through his trunk which he first noticed in 2013 (Fig. 10.1). He also noticed about 10 lb of weight loss. A skin biopsy from left chest wall was performed in October of 2014 and histopathologic finding was consistent with urticaria pigmentosa. Peripheral blood counts were normal. The bone marrow biopsy in April 2014 showed normocellular bone marrow with involvement by SM (spindle-shaped mast cells with aberrant CD25 expression comprising less than 5% of cellularity) and normal trilineage hematopoiesis. *KIT D816V* was detected by NGS at a variable allele frequency of 7.4%. There was no hepatosplenomegaly on imaging. He also had elevated serum tryptase levels which was 68.4 µg/L in March 2018. He was started on midostaurin 50 mg twice daily starting October 2018. His pruritus and skin rash improved. Serum tryptase levels are still elevated and was 303 µg/L in May 2020. He is tolerating midostaurin well except for nausea managed with antiemetics.

Indolent SM is the second most common form of SM in adults. The term ISM is used for patients with SM without an associated hematologic neoplasm and with <20% mast cells in the bone marrow, low mast cell/disease burden (defined as ≤ 1 "B findings" as per Table 10.3), and no organ dysfunction (defined as no "C findings" as per Table 10.3). Mast cell infiltrates may be detected in various organs (including liver, spleen, and gastrointestinal tract) in ISM, but by definition there is no organ dysfunction. Otherwise, the diagnosis would be ASM. If ≥ 2 "B findings"

Fig. 10.1 Urticaria pigmentosa rash in a patient with ISM

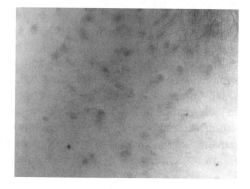

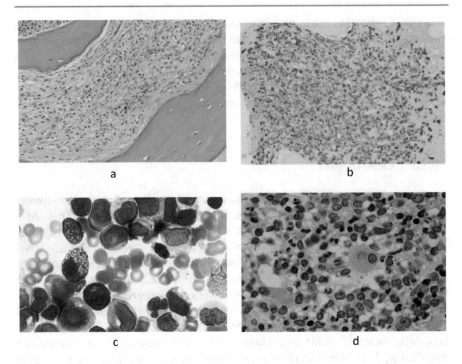

Fig. 10.2 Bone marrow features of SM. **a** Bone marrow biopsy from a patient with ISM showing dense paratrabecular aggregates of spindle-shaped mast cells. Osteosclerosis is evident. Such aggregates fulfill the major WHO criteria for SM. **b** Immunohistochemistry for mast cell tryptase highlights the mast cell aggregates. **c** SM-AHN. Bone marrow aspirate showing increased mast cells and myeloblasts in a case of SM associated with MDS with excess blasts-2. **d** Bone marrow biopsy from SM associated with MDS showing dysplastic megakaryocytes and myeloid precursors

are present, the diagnosis changes to smoldering SM. The clinical course is generally indolent, though severe anaphylaxis can be seen more often compared to more aggressive forms of SM. The *KIT* D816V mutation is detected in >90% of ISM cases, with other *KIT* mutations detected in a portion of the remaining patients upon sequencing of the *KIT* gene.

Case 2 has the typical presentation with urticaria pigmentosa dominating the clinical picture. The patient did not have features related to other organ dysfunction from mast cell infiltration (C findings). Therefore, he would be expected to have a prolonged indolent clinical course and focus of therapy would be to manage symptoms as well as prevent mast cell proliferation. Therapy directed at KIT D816V mutation is appropriate in this case given the dominant role of this mutation in pathogenesis of ISM. Although he responded well to midostaurin clinically with significant improvement in skin rash, this was not reflected in tryptase level which remained high. Therefore, it appears that tryptase level alone cannot be used to follow response of SM to KIT-directed therapy and response should be assessed by a combination of clinical as well as pathologic features. Gastrointestinal side effects from midostaurin can be significant and may require supportive management as in this case.

10.4 Clinical Features of SM

The clinical features of SM result from release of mast cell mediators, infiltration of organs, or the associated neoplasm in case of SM-AHN. Constitutional symptoms like fever, night sweats, and weight loss are common. Mediators induce a wide array of allergic-type symptoms including urticaria, episodic flushing, hypotension, tachycardia, and bronchospasm [18]. The classic clinical finding of indolent forms of SM is skin infiltration with mast cells manifesting as urticaria pigmentosa which is a common presenting feature (Fig. 10.1). Patients may have bone lesions on X-ray which includes osteosclerosis, osteoporosis, or lytic lesions and pathologic fractures may occur. Hepatosplenomegaly is not uncommon, however lymphadenopathy is rare. Bone marrow involvement may manifest as peripheral blood cytopenia which could be from mast cell infiltration or from the associated AHN. Gastrointestinal symptoms include abdominal pain, nausea, diarrhea, and heartburn and does not always denote infiltration of gastrointestinal tract with mast cells. Neurologic symptoms of headache, cognitive impairment, and depression have been observed [18]. In the case of SM-AHN, symptoms of mediator release as well as urticaria pigmentosa and other organ infiltration are unusual and the diagnosis is often made concurrently with or during the course of treatment of the associated hematologic neoplasm, most commonly AML or MDS.

Laboratory studies for serum tryptase level are helpful in the initial diagnostic work-up. In SM, a persistently elevated serum tryptase level (>20 ng/ml) is a minor diagnostic criterion as per the WHO [1]. The levels vary according to the type of SM; a greater proportion of ASM and SM-AHN patients exhibit a markedly elevated serum tryptase level (>200 ng/ml) compared to the ISM. Levels over 200 ng/ml are also seen in smoldering SM which is characterized by a higher mast cell burden compared to ISM [15]. However, serum tryptase levels are not specific to SM and may be elevated in the presence of other myeloid neoplasms such as AML, MDS, and CML. In the absence of another myeloid malignancy, serum tryptase is a relatively specific marker for mast cell burden. In reactive mast cell activation, serum tryptase is elevated during and within several hours of the patient's symptoms but returns to a normal level when the patient is asymptomatic, indicating an episode of mast cell activation without an increase in total body mast cell number. On the other hand, persistent elevation of baseline serum total tryptase >20 ng/mL drawn while the patient is asymptomatic indicates an increase in total body mast cell number. If baseline tryptase is elevated on two occasions, an evaluation for SM should be pursued.

10.5 Treatment of SM

The goals of treatment in SM are to improve mediator release symptoms as well as to decrease mast cell burden in order to improve urticaria pigmentosa rash and other organ dysfunction if present. In the case of SM-AHN, the primary goal is to treat the AHN.

Attempts have been made to develop prognostic scoring systems for SM based on clinical, laboratory, and molecular features. Details of these scoring systems have been published elsewhere [15]. Some of the adverse prognostic factors include age over 60 years and elevated alkaline phosphatase level (for non-advanced SM), and anemia, thrombocytopenia, high tryptase level, lack of skin involvement as well as presence of high-risk mutations in genes including *ASXL1, RUNX1, DNMT3A, SRSF2,* and *NRAS* [15]. These mutations are a feature of advanced forms of SM including SM-AHN where the AHN determines prognosis.

Given the universal presence of *KIT* mutation in SM and its role as the primary driver of mast cell proliferation and survival, KIT inhibitors are the logical choice to lower mast cell burden. Midostaurin (PKC 412) a multikinase inhibitor with known targets including *FLT3 and KIT* was evaluated for SM. The phase II trial of midostaurin in advanced SM showed an overall response rate (ORR) of 60% and a major response was seen in 45% of patients. Complete remissions, however, were not observed [20]. Based on these results, midostaurin received FDA approval for advanced SM. The more selective KIT inhibitor avapritinib (BLU 285) is a potent inhibitor of D816-mutated KIT and has shown higher response rate than midostaurin in an ongoing Phase 1 study although it must be pointed out that the responses were assessed by different criteria. The ORR for avapritinib was 77% which included 13% CR and CR with partial hematologic recovery [21]. Response to therapy in the avapritinib trial was assessed by the stringent International Working Group— Myeloproliferative neoplasms Research and Treatment and the European Competence Network on Mastocytosis criteria where a CR was defined as resolution of all symptoms and end-organ damage with blood counts as follows: ANC >1 x 10^9/l with normal differential, hemoglobin level 11 g/dl, and platelet count (100 x 10^9/l), resolution of hepatosplenomegaly and other end-organ damage, a tryptase level less than 20 ng/ml, and resolution of neoplastic cells in the bone marrow or organ of known involvement [22]. Midostaurin and avapritinib are FDA approved for advanced SM. Gastrointestinal side effects, fatigue, and edema are commonly observed side effects with these agents and often requires dose reduction.

In the very rare situation where D816 mutation in *KIT* is not detected, it is important to sequence other exons of the *KIT* gene for mutations in its extracellular, transmembrane, or juxtamembrane domains since some of these mutations are sensitive to imatinib which can induce clinical response in such cases [18]. Cladribine has been used in advanced SM and has an ORR of around 50% with a higher response rate in more indolent forms of SM [18, 23]. It may be a choice for patients who fail KIT inhibitor therapy or need more rapid debulking of mast cell burden. Interferon alpha in combination with corticosteroids has also shown activity in SM but this therapy has more side effects and poor tolerability [18, 24].

Relief of symptoms due to mediator release can be addressed by histamine receptor blockers, corticosteroids, cromolyn sodium, and leukotriene antagonists. Treatment of osteoporosis with biphosphonates has also been recommended [18, 19].

Majority of patients with advanced SM have associated AHN and curative therapy for the AHN by allogeneic hematopoietic stem cell transplantation (allo-HSCT) is the preferred approach in suitable candidates. Allo-HSCT for ASM has been attempted as a potentially curative therapy for patients with advanced SM. There are no randomized studies to show benefit and the largest experience is from a retrospective series of 57 patients with following SM subtypes: SM-AHN (38 patients), MCL (12 patients), and ASM (7 patients). The overall survival at 3 years was 57% but depended on type of SM (MCL: 17%, ASM: 43%, SM-AHN: 74%). Diagnosis of MCL and use of reduced intensity conditioning were associated with worse outcomes after HSCT [25]. The role and timing of allo-HSCT, as well as optimal conditioning regimen, remain to be clarified in other forms of advanced SM besides SM-AHN [26]. It is important to recognize that in case of SM-AHN, the residual bone marrow mast cell infiltrate may persist after successful allo-HSCT and does not mean failure of HSCT provided there is no evidence of the AHN.

References

1. Swerdlow SH et al (2017) WHO classification of tumours of haematopoietic and lymphoid tissues, revised 4th edn. International Agency for Research on Cancer, Lyon, France
2. Nagata H, Worobec AS, Oh CK et al (1995) Identification of a point mutation in the catalytic domain of the protooncogene c-kit in peripheral blood mononuclear cells of patients who have mastocytosis with an associated hematologic disorder. Proc Natl Acad Sci U S A 92:10560
3. Ustun C, Arock M, Kluin-Nelemans HC et al (2016) Advanced systemic mastocytosis: from molecular and genetic progress to clinical practice. Haematologica 101(10):1133–1143
4. Schaab J, Schnittger S. Sotlar K et al (2013) Comprehensive mutational profiling in advanced systemic Mastocytosis. Blood 12(14):460–466
5. Jawhar M, Schwaab J, Schnittger S et al (2016) Additional mutations in SRSF2, ASXL1 and or RUNX1identify a high risk group of patients with KIT D816V(+) advances systemic mastocytosis. Leukemia 30(1):136–143
6. Jawhar m, Schwaab J, Schnittger S et al (2015) Molecular profiling of myeloid progenitor cells in multimutated advanced systemic mastocytosis identifies KITD8116V as a distinct and late event Leukmaia 29(5):1115–1122
7. Hanssens K, Brenet F, Agopian J et al (2014) SRSF2-p95 hotspot mutation is hifhly associated with advanced forms of mastocytosis and mutations in epigenetic regulator genes. Haematologica 99(5):830–835
8. Yavuz AS, Lipsky PE, Yavuz S et al (2002) Evidence for the involvement of a hematopoietic progenitor cell in systemic mastocytosis from single-cell analysis of mutations in the c-kit gene. Blood 100:661
9. Grootens J, Ungerstedt JS, Ekoff M et al (2019) Single cell analysis reveals the KIT D816V mutation in hematopoietic stem and progenitor cells in systemic mastocytosis. EBioMedicine 43:150–158
10. Naumann N, Jawhar M, Schwaab J (2018) Incidence and prognostic impact of cytogenetic aberrations in patients with systemic Mastocytosis. Genes Chromosomes Cancer 57(5):252–259

11. Pullarkat V, Bedell V, Kim Y et al (2007) Neoplastic mast cells in systemic mastocytosis associated with t(8;21) acute myeloid leukemia are derived from the leukemic clone. Leuk Res 31(2):261–265
12. Pullarkat VA, Bueso-Ramos C, Lai R et al (2003) Systemic mastocytosis associated with clonal hematological non mast cell lineage disease: analysis of clinicopathologic features and activating c-kit mtations. Am J Hematol 73(1):12–17
13. Morgado JM, Perbellini O, Johnson RC et al (2013) CD30 expression by bone marrow mast cells from different diagnostic variants of systemic mastocytosis. Histopathology 63:780–787
14. Sotlar K, Cerny-Reiterer S, Petat-Dutter K et al (2011) Aberrant expression of CD30 in neoplastic mast cells in high-grade mastocytosis. Mod Pathol 24:585–595
15. Reiter A, George TI, Gotlib J (2020) New developments in diagnosis, prognostication and treatment of advanced systemic mastocytosis. Blood 35(16):1365–1376
16. Kim Y, Weiss LM, Chen YY, Pullarkat V (2007) Distinct clonal origins of systemic mastocytosis and associated B-cell lymphoma. Leuk Res 31(12):1749–1754
17. Johnson RC, Savage NM, Chiang T et al (2013) Hidden mastocytosis in acute myeloid leukemia with t(8;21)(q22;q22). Am J Clin Pathol 140(4):525–535
18. Pardanani A (2019) Systemic mastocytosis in adults: 2019 update on diagnosis, risk stratification and management. Am J Hematol 94:363–377
19. Pardanani A (2013) How I treat patients with indolent and smoldering mastocytosis (rare conditions but difficult to manage). Blood 121:3085–3094
20. Gotlib J, Kluin-Nelemans HC, George TI et al (2016) Efficacy and safety of midostaurin in advanced systemic mastocytosis. N Engl J Med 374:2530–2541
21. Radia D, Deininger M, Gotlib J et al (2019) Avapritinib, a potent and selective inhibitor of KIT D816V induces complete and durable responses in patients with advanced systemic mastocytosis European Hematology Association Congress. Amsterdam, The Netherlands
22. Gotlib J, Pardanani A, Akin C et al (2013) International working group-myeloproliferative neoplasms research and treatment (IWG-MRT) & European competence network on mastocytosis (ECNM) consensus response criteria in advanced systemic mastocytosis. Blood 121
23. Kluin –Nelemans C, Oldhoff JM, Van Doormaal JJ (2003) Cladaribine therapy for systemic mastocytosis. Blood 102: 4270–4276
24. Casassus P, Caillat-Vigneron N, Martin A et al (2002) Treatment of adult systemic mastocytosis with interferon-alpha: results of a multicentre phase II trial on 20 patients. Br J Haematol 119:1090–1097
25. Ustin C, Reiter A, Scott BL (2014) Hematopoietic stem cell transplantation for advanced systemic mastocytosis. J Clin Oncol 32:3264–3274
26. Ustun C, Gotlib J, Popat U et al (2016) Consensus opinion on allogeneic hematopoietuc cell transplantation in advanced systemic mastocytosis. Biol Blood Marrow Transplant 22:1348–1356

Chimeric Antigen Receptor (CAR) T Cell Therapy for B-Acute Lymphoblastic Leukemia (B-ALL)

11

Geoffrey Shouse, Elizabeth Budde, and Stephen Forman

Contents

11.1 CASE 1: *CAR-T Cell Therapy for Refractory/Relapsed B-ALL with Extramedullary Disease*

A 25-year-old female with Philadelphia chromosome negative B-ALL was evaluated for salvage therapy with CD19-directed CAR-T cell therapy. She was diagnosed with ALL with MLL rearrangement 3 years previously. At diagnosis, she did not have CNS involvement. HLA typing revealed her sister was histocompatible.

G. Shouse (✉) · E. Budde · S. Forman
Department of Hematology and Hematopoietic Cell Transplantation, City of Hope National
Medical Center, 1500 E Duarte Rd., Duarte, CA 91010, USA
e-mail: gshouse@coh.org

E. Budde
e-mail: ebudde@coh.org

S. Forman
e-mail: SForman@coh.org

© Springer Nature Switzerland AG 2021
V. Pullarkat and G. Marcucci (eds.), *Biology and Treatment of Leukemia and Bone Marrow Neoplasms*, Cancer Treatment and Research 181,
https://doi.org/10.1007/978-3-030-78311-2_11

She was in a minimal residual disease (MRD) positive morphologic remission after induction on a pediatric regimen. She remained MRD positive after consolidation and was subsequently treated with the CD19-CD3 bispecific antibody blinatumomab, which converted her to an MRD negative remission after one cycle. Her course was complicated by neurotoxicity. She had subsequent consolidation with a matched related allogeneic stem cell transplant (allo-HCT) from her sister after myeloablative conditioning using fractionated total body irradiation and etoposide. Unfortunately, despite adequate CNS prophylaxis, she developed a relapse in her optic nerve. She was treated with radiation and intrathecal chemotherapy but developed subsequent leptomeningeal relapse. She had an Ommaya reservoir placed and received CNS radiation and intrathecal chemotherapy. Subsequently, she had MRD relapse in the bone marrow with CNS relapse again and was treated with blinatumomab. After one cycle, she was once again in MRD negative remission, but at cycle 5 she relapsed again in the CNS. At that time, she was treated with CD19-directed CAR-T cell therapy. Her post infusion course was complicated by grade 3 neurotoxicity which resolved after corticosteroids. She was once again in MRD negative remission after CAR-T cell therapy and has remained disease free for more than 18 months.

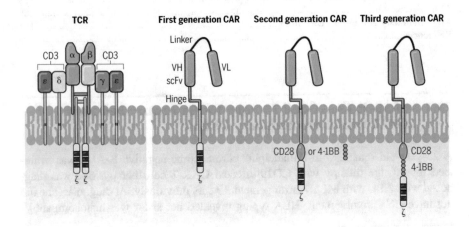

Fig. 11.1 Engineered T cells: design of TCR versus CAR-T cells. T cells can be redirected to have specificity for tumors by the introduction of (**left**) transgenic TCRs (T cell receptors) or (**right**) CAR proteins. CARs are fusion proteins composed of an extracellular portion that is usually derived from an antibody and intracellular signaling molecules derived from T cell signaling proteins. First-generation CARs contain CD3ζ whereas second-generation CARs consist of two costimulatory domains linked to CD3ζ. scFv, single-chain variable fragment; VH, variable heavy chain; VL, variable light chain. Figure [2] Adapted from CAR-T cell immunotherapy for human cancer, June et al 2018, AAAS. Reprinted with permission from AAAS, copyright 2018 by AAAS

11.2 Discussion

What are CAR-T cells?

Chimeric Antigen Receptor T (CAR-T) cells are a form of adoptive immunotherapy in which T cells are collected, genetically manipulated in vitro, and then introduced into the patient. The manipulation involves transduction of a genetic construct designed to express a novel transmembrane protein, the chimeric antigen receptor (CAR) [1]. This chimeric protein is designed to have several domains in order to achieve tumor antigen specificity, adequate stimulation, and T cell activation. A prototypical CAR protein is depicted in Fig. 11.1, which has been reproduced from a prior publication with permission [2]. The extracellular antigen recognition domain is typically designed utilizing an immunoglobulin single-chain variable region known to recognize and bind a target protein [1]. In the case of CAR-T cells for ALL, this target protein most often is CD19. The rationale for CD19 as a target comes from several facts including its near-universal expression in B-ALL, its high level of expression on B cells, and its specificity and restricted expression mainly to B cells and not other cells or tissues in the body [3]. Additional CAR-T cell domains include the hinge region, the transmembrane domain, and the intracellular T cell stimulatory domain. The stimulatory domain is typically derived from the CD3ζ molecule, the function of which is to activate the T cell in response to CAR binding to the target protein. Early studies with CAR-T cells demonstrated increased efficacy with the presence of costimulatory domains within the CAR molecules [4–10]. As such, second-generation CAR-T cells are designed to also contain a second intracellular domain that acts as a co-stimulator. These are typically derived from the CD28 molecule or 4-1BB. Additional domains may include linkers, such as a portion of the epidermal growth factor receptor, for which there is a humanized antibody. The rationale for this linker being that if it became necessary to remove or inactivate the CAR-T cells within a short time period, inactivating antibodies targeting the linker region could be utilized. In this way, there is a backup in place to control CAR-T cell function in the case of toxicity. Once joined together, these domains make up the CAR gene. Once it is constructed, the chimeric antigen receptor gene is transduced into T cells, typically with the use of viral vectors. After generation of the CAR expressing T cells, they are expanded and transfused into the patient.

What is the indication for CAR-T cells in patients with ALL?

Tisagenlecleucel is an autologous CAR-T cell product designed to target CD19 and is approved by the United States Food and Drug Administration (FDA) for the treatment of patients that are aged 25 or younger with B cell precursor acute lymphoblastic leukemia that is refractory or in second or later relapse [11]. It is currently the only FDA-approved CAR-T cell therapeutic approved for ALL at this time.

How are CAR-T cells manufactured and administered?

The T cell collection and modification process can vary to some degree, depending on the specifications of the manufacturing site. This process has been reviewed previously [12–15]. Several steps are employed, however, regardless of this variability. For autologous CAR-T products, first, T cells are collected from the patient through leukapheresis. Second, the collected bulk T cells may be enriched or purified further. Next, the T cells are activated in culture using cytokines or other similar techniques. The CAR transgene is then introduced into the T cells. These T cells are then cultured further and expanded. Finally, the cells are reintroduced into the patient [12, 14, 16]. Prior to infusion of the CAR-T cell product, however, patients are typically treated with lymphodepleting chemotherapy. The combination of fludarabine and cyclophosphamide is commonly used. The idea behind this step is to remove inhibitory endogenous T regulatory cells, allowing enhanced activation and propagation of the CAR-T cells. Several studies indicate this step is critical to increase CAR-T cell expansion, increase serum CAR-T cell peak numbers, enhance response rates to CAR-T cells as well as improve long-term survival [17–21]. Of note, however, lymphodepleting chemotherapy is also associated with increased toxicity, with reportedly higher rates of cytokine release syndrome (CRS) and cytokine-related encephalopathy syndrome (CRES) [20, 22]. After T cell infusion, patients are typically kept in the hospital for a period of time for close monitoring for toxicity.

What is the efficacy of CAR-T cell therapy in B-ALL?

The efficacy of CD19-directed CAR-T cell therapy has been demonstrated in B cell malignancies in several early trials [23–28]. In addition, several larger trials have evaluated the efficacy of CD19-directed CAR-T cell therapy in B cell ALL with response rates as high as 90% [29–31]. A single institution study demonstrated an 83% CR rate in 53 adult patients with heavily pretreated relapsed or refractory B cell ALL age 23–74 [29]. Patients with lower disease burden tended to have more lasting remissions and better outcomes [event-free survival (EFS) 11 months, overall survival (OS) >20 months] compared to patients with higher disease burden or extramedullary disease (OS 12 months). In addition, the only currently FDA-approved CAR-T cell product, tisagenlecleucel, was evaluated for overall remission rate in a multi-center phase 2 study in children and young adults with relapsed or refractory, CD19 positive, B cell ALL [30]. 75 patients received infusion of the autologous CAR-T cell product and were evaluated for efficacy. The primary endpoint, overall remission rate at 3 months, was 81%. Importantly, all patients achieving remission were negative for MRD. EFS was 73% at 6 months and dropped to 50% at 12 months, while OS was 76% at 12 months.

Are CAR-T cells effective for CNS disease and/or extramedullary disease?

Several lines of evidence indicate a role for CAR-T cell therapy for CNS relapses of B-ALL. First, it has been demonstrated in several studies that CAR-T cells are capable of penetrating the central nervous system and CAR-T cells have been detected in the CNS [28, 32, 33]. In addition, CAR-T cell therapy has proven efficacious at clearing CNS relapses and preventing CNS recurrence. For example, in an NCI study, the two patients with known CNS disease had clearance after

CD19-directed CAR-T cell infusion [28]. Additionally, in a study by the University of Pennsylvania, 12 patients with known CNS disease had clearance of their leukemia and overall remission after CAR-T cell therapy [33]. Four patients ended up relapsing, but their CNS remained free of disease.

Extramedullary disease, especially extramedullary relapse after allo-HCT, confers a dire prognosis in B-ALL. There is currently no standard therapy, although combinations of chemotherapy, immunotherapy, stem cell transplant, radiation, and other therapies have been attempted. There is a relative paucity of studies investigating this particular disease site; however, seven patients on an early phase trial and additional published cases have demonstrated the efficacy of CD19-directed CAR-T cell therapy in extramedullary B-ALL, even in extramedullary relapse after allo-HCT [34–36]. Although no large controlled studies have been published on this topic to date, these preliminary reports are encouraging in this subset of patients with limited effective treatment options.

11.3 CASE 2: *Identification and Management of CAR-T Cell Toxicities*

A 20-year-old male was diagnosed with B-ALL at age 7. He was treated to remission with a pediatric protocol and relapsed 1 year after completing his therapy. He achieved a second remission only to relapse again 4 years later. At that time, he had salvage chemotherapy followed by matched related sibling allo-HCT. Six months after the transplant he developed a CNS only relapse that was treated with radiation and intrathecal chemotherapy. He then developed a systemic relapse that was refractory to donor lymphocyte infusion and he relapsed in the CNS again as well shortly after that. He was treated with blinatumomab and additional donor lymphocyte infusions for salvage therapy and achieved remission. Subsequently, he relapsed again in the CNS and at a low level in the bone marrow as well. He was treated with CD19-directed CAR-T cell therapy. Four days after CAR-T cell infusion, the patient developed high fevers up to 39.4 degrees Celsius. He developed hypotension that initially responded to IV fluid hydration but subsequently required vasopressor support. He received two doses of tocilizumab at 8 mg/kg IV and his fevers subsided and blood pressure normalized. At 8 days after the CAR-T cell infusion, the patient was noted to no longer be able to write a sentence, he was confused and unable to answer questions or follow commands. Neurologic work-up including brain MRI and EEG showed no evidence of etiology and the patient was initiated on dexamethasone 10 mg IV with rapid improvement of his neurologic status back to baseline. He was subsequently tapered off of the corticosteroids without event.

11.4 Discussion

What are the common toxicities of CAR-T cells?

CAR-T cell therapy has a toxicity profile that is unique and can differ to some extent in severity based on factors like the design of the CAR itself, target of the CAR-T cell, the T cell source, as well as other factors. As such, the toxicity profile of a particular CAR-T construct as well as the risk of development of various toxicities can be somewhat difficult to judge. Despite this fact, several common toxicities have been documented in ALL patients and patients with other B cell malignancies treated with CD19-directed CAR-T cell therapy. The two most common toxicities to date have consisted of cytokine release syndrome (CRS) and neurotoxicity, sometimes referred to as CAR-T-related encephalopathy syndrome (CRES) or immune effector cell-associated neurotoxicity syndrome (ICANS). The nomenclature and grading of these toxicities have been evolving over the last several years. In an effort to standardize these toxicities, the American Society of Transplant and Cellular Therapy (ASTCT) facilitated a meeting of experts from multiple centers including representatives from the Center for International Blood and Marrow Transplant Research (CIBMTR), the American Society of Hematology (ASH), and the National Cancer Institute (NCI). This meeting published approved consensus recommendations for the naming and grading of CRS and neurotoxicity associated with immune effector cells [37].

In clinical trials utilizing CD19-directed CAR-T cell therapy, the most commonly reported toxicity was CRS, reportedly occurring as frequently as 74–100% of the time [22, 30, 38, 39]. The pathogenesis is thought to involve a process catalyzed initially by the release of effector cytokines by activated CAR-T cells

Table 11.1 Signs and symptoms of CRS

Organ system	Signs/symptoms
Constitutional	Fever, rigors, malaise, fatigue, anorexia, arthralgias
Cardiovascular	Tachycardia, widened pulse pressure, hypotension, arrhythmias, decreased LV EF, elevated cardiac enzymes, prolonged QT interval
Gastrointestinal	Nausea, emesis, diarrhea, transaminitis, hyperbilirubinemia
Hematologic	Pancytopenia, B cell aplasia, prolonged prothrombin and activated partial thromboplastin time, elevated D-dimer, hypofibrinogenemia, disseminated intravascular coagulation, hemophagocytic lymphohistiocytosis
Musculoskeletal	Myalgias, elevated creatine kinase, generalized weakness
Neurologic	Headaches, altered level of consciousness, delirium, aphasia, agraphia, ataxia, tremor, myoclonus, seizures
Pulmonary	Tachypnea, hypoxia, capillary leak
Renal	Acute kidney injury, hyponatremia, hypokalemia, hypophosphatemia, tumor lysis syndrome

Table 11.2 CRS grading, [35] Adapted from the CTCAE consensus guidelines

CRS parameter	Grade 1	Grade 2	Grade 3	Grade 4
Fever	Temp. ≥ 38 ° C	Temp. ≥ 38 ° C	Temp. ≥ 38 °C with	Temp. ≥ 38 °C
Hypotension	None	Not requiring vasopressors and/or	Requiring vasopressor with or without vasopressin and/or	Requiring multiple vasopressors (excluding vasopressin)
Hypoxia	None	Requiring low-flow nasal cannula or blow-by (≤ 6L/minute)	Requiring high-flow nasal cannula, facemask, nonrebreather mask, or Venturi mask	Requiring positive pressure ventilation (e.g., CPAP, BiPAP, intubation, and mechanical ventilation)

upon their recognition of target. Cytokines implicated include interleukin-2, interferon gamma, and tumor necrosis factor- alpha. This in turn leads to an overproduction of cytokines, including interleukin- 6, interleukin- 10, among others, by macrophages and endothelial cells as well as various additional immune and other cell types leading to a systemic inflammatory response. The ASTCT defines CRS as "a supraphysiologic response following any immune therapy that results in the activation or engagement of endogenous or infused T cells and/or immune effector cells. Symptoms can be progressive, must include fever at the onset, and may include hypotension, capillary leak (hypoxia) and end organ dysfunction" [37].

Signs and symptoms of CRS demonstrate involvement of multiple organ systems and can range from mild, which include fever, myalgias, fatigue, mild hypotension, to severe symptoms, including respiratory failure, coagulopathy, and multi-organ failure, summarized in Table 11.1. Laboratory tests may demonstrate elevation of inflammatory markers including C-reactive protein (CRP) and ferritin and in more severe cases, evidence of end organ damage may be evidenced by rising serum creatinine, bilirubin, or liver enzymes. The onset of symptoms typically occurs within 1–5 days of T cell infusion and commonly is heralded by fevers.

Several grading systems have been employed previously including the National Cancer Institute Common Terminology Criteria for Adverse events (CTCAE) v4.03 [40] and v5.0 [41], other criteria proposed by Lee et al. [42], criteria proposed by the Memorial Sloan Kettering Cancer Center [29], the CARTOX criteria published by the MD Anderson Cancer Center CAR-T Therapy-Associated Toxicity Working Group [43], and the Penn Criteria [44] published by the University of Pennsylvania. Each of these grading systems had benefits and drawbacks. The use of various grading systems in different CAR-T trials made the uniform implementation of a single grading system that could guide therapeutic intervention more difficult. In an attempt to address this, as discussed above, the grading system published by the ASTCT in 2018 as part of a consensus statement meant to make identification and

Table 11.3 ICANS grading, [35] Adapted from the CTCAE consensus guidelines

Neurotoxicity domain	Grade 1	Grade 2	Grade 3	Grade 4
ICE score	7–9	3–6	0–2	0 (patient is unarousable, unable to perform ICE)
Depressed level of consciousness	Awakens spontaneously	Awakens to voice	Awakens only to tactile stimulus	Patient unarousable or requires vigorous repetitive tactile stimuli to arouse Stupor or coma
Seizure	N/A	N/A	Any clinical seizure that resolves rapidly or nonconvulsive seizure on EEG that resolves with intervention	Life-threatening prolonged seizure (>5 min), or repetitive clinical or electrical seizures without return to baseline
Motor findings	N/A	N/A	N/A	Deep focal motor weakness such as hemiparesis or paraparesis
Elevated ICP/cerebral edema	N/A	N/A	Focal/local edema on neuroimaging	Diffuse cerebral edema on neuroimaging, decerebrate, or decorticate posturing; cranial nerve VI palsy; papilledema; or Cushing's triad

treatment of CAR-T-related toxicities more uniform and simplified. In this system, for CRS grading, there is a distinction between fever (required for all grades), hypotension requiring vasopressors (grade 3 or 4), or amounts of supplemental oxygen (grade 2 is low flow, grade 3 is high flow, grade 4 is positive pressure) to note grades 1–4, summarized in Table 11.2 [37]. The management of these toxicities will be discussed below.

Neurotoxicity is another common toxicity associated with CAR-T cell therapy. It is not completely unique to this type of adoptive immunotherapy, however, so broader terms have been used to identify this syndrome. These have included CAR-T-related encephalopathy syndrome (CRES) and immune effector cell-associated neurotoxicity syndrome (ICANS) [37, 43]. Although related to CRS, this syndrome can appear independently of CRS and has a timing of onset that is distinct as well. It can reportedly occur any time after CAR-T cell infusion and can occur before, during, after, or even in the absence of CRS. Symptoms include headache, seizures, delirium, anxiety, tremor, impaired writing ability, aphasia, decreased consciousness, and can progress to coma with cerebral edema. Many patients will have a stepwise progression of stereotypic symptoms presenting initially with tremor, dysgraphia, mild expressive aphasia, apraxia, mild lethargy, and impaired attention. The expressive aphasia appears to be a very specific symptom of neurotoxicity related to CAR-T cell therapy. In more severe cases, the aphasia can progress to global aphasia, where the patient is essentially mute and unable to follow commands, while still appearing awake. Lethargy may progress to frank coma. Rarely, cerebral edema may occur concurrently and can be fatal. ICANS grading is summarized in Table 11.3.

The underlying pathophysiology has yet to be elucidated, although several theories and preliminary evidence exist. There is suggestion of off target CAR-T activation within the CNS leading to production of cytokines within this domain. Other theories suggest that cytokines from the blood stream may disrupt the blood-brain barrier and also influence endothelial cells on the blood-brain barrier to secrete IL-6 [20]. Regardless of the etiology, the ASCTC consensus definition is as follows: "a disorder characterized by a pathologic process involving the central nervous system following any immune therapy that results in the activation or engagement of endogenous or infused T cells and/or other immune effector cells. Symptoms or signs can be progressive and may include aphasia, altered level of consciousness, impairment of cognitive skills, motor weakness, seizures, and cerebral edema" [37].

What are risk factors associated with the development of CRS?

Several factors have emerged as being potentially correlated with rates of toxicity after CAR-T cell therapy. Disease type tends to correlate with frequency of CRS with NHL rates (30–57%) being lower than those seen in ALL (74–100%) [45]. In addition, tumor burden correlated with rates of CRS and neurotoxicity. For example, ALL patients with >25% blasts in the bone marrow had significantly higher rates of CRS, while very low CRS rates were seen in patients with <5% bone marrow blasts [46]. Interestingly, lymphodepleting chemotherapy in these cases actually led to lower rates of CRS, suggesting a greater importance in the response to the bone marrow burden of disease rather than the increased toxicity seen from depletion of regulatory T cells. Additional factors related to development of CRS may include the epitope chosen on the target protein, composition of the T cell subpopulation, and the CAR-T cell dose and expansion peak. Despite this knowledge, it is difficult to predict if a patient will develop CRS or which patient will develop severe CRS. Most available biomarkers that can be measured in real time, including CRP and ferritin, tend to increase simultaneously with worsening CRS, rather than antecedently, making them poor markers for CRS severity prediction [46].

How is CRS managed after CAR-T cell administration?

Although there are no consensus guidelines to guide the therapy for CRS, some practical experience from prior clinical trials as well as experts in the field can provide some assistance. Once CRS is suspected, typically due to the presence of fevers after CAR-T cell administration, it is important to rule out other causes of fever, such as infection, particularly since many of these patients will be neutropenic. A thorough history and physical examination with tailored laboratory testing, including blood cultures, should be performed with additional testing as clinically indicated. Supportive measures should be initiated in the presence of more severe CRS symptoms such as addition of supplemental oxygen for hypoxemia or fluid resuscitation for hypotension. Monitoring in the ICU and use of vasopressors or positive pressure ventilation for rapidly progressive or severe CRS should be performed as indicated. Typically, stable grade 1 CRS can be monitored, while more severe CRS with demonstration of end organ damage, or rapidly worsening CRS should be treated. The IL-6 receptor antagonist, tocilizumab, has been utilized extensively to ameliorate CRS toxicities after CAR-T cell infusions in several trials [17, 26–28, 32, 47]. Evidence indicates that use of tocilizumab does not affect CAR-T cell efficacy in patients with B cell ALL [28, 32]. Based on these published experiences, tocilizumab has gained FDA approval for use in CAR-T-related CRS. The recommended dosing for tocilizumab varies from 4 to 8 mg/kg with a capped dose of 800 mg total per dose. Repeat dosing can be given every 8 h up to 3 doses. If no improvement is seen, or the CRS continues to progress despite tocilizumab, additional interventions should be sought, including consideration of corticosteroids [26, 42]. There is no consensus on which corticosteroid is most efficacious, however most commonly dexamethasone is utilized.

There is some evidence to suggest that the use of corticosteroids may negatively influence the efficacy and persistence of CAR-T cells [23, 26], despite this fact, they have been used to effectively treat the toxicities of CRS in several studies [23, 26–28, 47, 48]. Given the potential for disrupting CAR-T cell therapeutic efficacy, their use for CRS is typically reserved for patients who fail to respond to tocilizumab. Other agents that can be considered for use in management of CRS toxicity include drugs that target IL-6, such as siltuximab [49], as well as those that target other cytokines, including infliximab [42], etanercept [17, 27, 42], and anakinra [42]. To date, there is no clear evidence to guide use of one agent over another.

How is neurotoxicity managed after CAR-T cell administration?

As discussed above, although there may be some overlap between CRS and neurotoxicity after CAR-T cell infusions, they do appear to be different syndromes. As such, the therapies and interventions differ. In addition, it is important to remain vigilant for neurotoxicity even after CRS is resolved or in the absence of CRS as it can occur independently. There is some evidence that neurotoxicity is mediated by CNS production of cytokines. These may be due to the presence of CAR-T cells in the CNS, as it has been previously shown that CAR-T cells can enter the CNS and are effective at treating CNS involvement by leukemia and preventing CNS relapse [17, 27, 28, 32, 50, 51]. In addition, there may be a role for IL-6 as well, given that high levels of IL-6 were identified in the CSF of patients experiencing neurotoxicity [42]. The use of tocilizumab in the treatment of neurotoxicity is questionable for two important reasons. First, the drug is thought to not be able to pass into the CNS [52]. As such, it is not able to influence the cytokines in that compartment. Second, tocilizumab is a monoclonal antibody against the IL-6 receptor, rather than the cytokine itself. As such, there is some evidence that levels of IL-6 may actually increase after tocilizumab administration [53]. Corticosteroids have shown excellent efficacy in ameliorating the neurotoxicity of CAR-T cell therapy. Dexamethasone is commonly utilized, given its excellent CNS penetration. Given the potential to compromise the efficacy of the CAR-T cells, it is typically withheld unless the neurotoxicity is beyond grade 2.

It is important to keep in mind that there may be other etiologies of neurotoxicity in patients being treated with CAR-T cell therapy. As such, a thorough work-up should be performed, including neurology consultation, brain imaging, and CSF sampling as clinically indicated. Evaluation for occult seizure activity with EEG monitoring and utilization of anti-epileptics may also be indicated.

11.5 CASE 3: *Sequencing CAR-T Cell Therapy with Other Treatments for Refractory/Relapsed B- ALL*

A 20-year-old male was diagnosed with Philadelphia chromosome like precursor B-ALL with a CRLF2 rearrangement at age 19. He was refractory to induction with a pediatric regimen. He had minimal response to salvage therapy with blinatumomab despite showing CD19 expression on his leukemic blasts. His blasts continued to express CD 19 and he was evaluated for CAR-T cell therapy. He tolerated the infusion and post-treatment period with minimal complications. He had grade 1 CRS and mild neurotoxicity that were managed supportively. After therapy, his bone marrow biopsy results indicated that he had achieved an MRD negative remission after CD19-directed CAR-T cell therapy. At 6 months post infusion, he developed MRD only relapse at a very low level detected by multi-parameter FLOW cytometry. He proceeded to allo-HCT with his matched sibling as donor and received myeloablative conditioning with FTBI and etoposide. His follow-up is ongoing at this time.

11.6 Discussion

What is the optimal timing of CAR-T cell therapy in relation to other treatments including stem cell transplant?

Despite the evidence of efficacy of CD19-directed CAR-T cell therapy in B-ALL, there are still many unanswered questions. Currently, adoptive immunotherapies, such as the CD19 bispecific T cell engager, blinatumomab, and immune targeted therapies, namely, the CD22 drug antibody conjugate inotuzumab, have shown promise in the relapsed and refractory setting. The optimal timing in relation to CAR-T cell therapy and effect on CAR-T cell efficacy have not been well studied to date. In a small case series, prior treatment with blinatumomab and/or inotuzumab did not appear to influence efficacy of CD19 CAR-T cell therapy [54]. One concern for using blinatumomab prior to CAR-T cell therapy would be the occurrence of CD19 negative relapse which would obviate the use of CD19-directed CAR-T cells. Additional studies are necessary to more clearly answer these questions, including investigation of the possibility of similar mechanisms of resistance to blinatumomab and CD19 CAR-T cell therapy given their overlapping mechanism of action.

Allo-HCT is a mainstay of consolidation therapy for patients with B-ALL in remission with intermediate and high risk for relapse. The optimal timing of CD19-directed CAR-T cell therapy in relation to allo-HCT remains incompletely elucidated [55, 56]. Some limited studies have reported no difference in outcomes of patients who relapsed after prior allo-HCT compared to those with no prior history of allo-HCT [56, 57]. These studies were not randomized or controlled and as such the published observations are useful for the design of future studies to more completely address this question. Despite the limitation, nothing appears to be lost by having prior allo-HCT before CAR-T cell therapy.

Prior to the advent of CAR-T cell therapy, outcomes for patients with B cell ALL that have relapsed after allo-HCT were dismal, with less than 10% remission rates, most of which were transient [58]. This group of patients, however, has excellent remission rates after CAR-T cell therapy. Majority of evidence suggests, however that for durable remission after CAR-T cell therapy, either long-lasting immune surveillance by the CAR-T cells must be present, or the patient must receive consolidation therapy with allo-HCT, in some cases a second or third transplant [55]. This topic is discussed further below.

Does CAR-T cell therapy require consolidation treatment with allo-HCT?

Allo-HCT represents a curative approach consolidation therapy for acute leukemia in patients with relapsed and high-risk disease. The effectiveness is due to a combination of both conditioning regimen and graft versus leukemia immune-mediated effects [59, 60]. The level of active disease burden at the time of transplant correlates with outcomes [61]. To this end, CAR-T cell therapy may represent an attractive approach for inducing MRD negative remission in preparation for allo-HCT. Several studies have indicated excellent outcomes utilizing this approach, even in the case of relapse after prior transplant [55]. But the question remains whether consolidation with allo-HCT is a requirement after CAR-T cell therapy for long-term remission.

Theoretically, long-term remission can be attained with the use of CAR-T cell therapy if long-term immune surveillance is maintained. This would require the persistence of CAR-T cells as well as persistence of expression of the CAR target on leukemic cells. Several determinants of CAR-T persistence have been described including the type of lymphodepleting chemotherapy [17, 62], the disease burden [17], and the CAR costimulatory domain [8]. The combination of fludarabine and cyclophosphamide was demonstrated to be superior to cyclophosphamide alone in terms of promoting durability and expansion of CAR-T cells as well as improving remission rates. The evidence of disease burden is not as clear-cut as only one study demonstrated more robust CAR-T cell proliferation in pediatric patients with higher blast counts. The costimulatory molecule, however, has the most robust effect on CAR-T cell persistence. For second-generation CARs, direct comparison of CD28-based CARs to those containing 41BB costimulatory molecules has shown that the presence of 41BB led to less cell exhaustion and a greater presence of central memory phenotype CAR-T cells as well as direct measurements of persistence in vivo [28, 32, 63, 64].

Even with the persistence of CAR-T cells in vivo, the expression of target protein on the leukemic cells must also be present for the CAR-T cells to remain effective. In fact, loss of CD19 expression, loss of the targeting epitope of CD19 by alternative splicing mutations, as well as phenotypic switch from ALL to AML are all mechanisms of leukemic escape from CAR-T therapy [32, 62, 65–73].

One potential method for overcoming the eventual acquired resistance to CAR-T cell therapy would be consolidation with allo-HCT. In this manner, a more diverse and responsive immune mechanism of surveillance could be employed by the donor immune cells to maintain longer remissions. Efficacy of this approach has been suggested by outcomes in several studies of patients treated with CAR-T cell therapy that ended up going on to allo-HCT compared to those that did not. It should also be noted that preliminary data suggest MRD negative remission prior to consolidation with allo-HCT is also a critical determinant of outcomes in this situation. For example, in a pediatric trial conducted at the NCI, 2 out of 21 patients treated to CR with CAR-T relapsed after consolidation with allo-HCT, while 6 out of 7 relapsed of those treated without allo-HCT [28, 74]. A similar trend was seen in patients treated on other studies as well [17, 28–30, 32, 34, 62, 74, 75].

11.7   Summary and Future Directions

CD19-directed CAR-T cell therapy represents a very efficacious, FDA-approved therapy for relapsed or refractory B cell acute lymphoblastic leukemia. CAR-T cell therapy has a diverse and variably severe set of toxicities and a trend toward a unified description, grading, and treatment of these toxicities is ongoing. Several resistance mechanisms exist allowing for relapse after CAR-T cell therapy. The optimal selection of patients for CAR-T cell therapy has not been completely elucidated and taking into consideration the factors specific to the disease as well as all other available therapies is important. Some of the challenges and drawbacks of CAR-T cell therapy, especially in B-ALL which can be a rapidly fatal disease, include the cost of the treatment as well as the time it takes for manufacturing the cells. This timeframe can take as long as 2–3 weeks in some instances, during which time the patient may have uncontrolled growth of disease. Ongoing studies include targeting of other leukemia molecules such as CD22, manipulation of CAR-T cells and CAR constructs, and combination of CAR-T therapy with other immunotherapies, among others. One interesting future direction involves the combination of two CAR-T populations targeted against both CD19 and CD22. In this way, it is thought the therapy may overcome the resistance brought about by loss of CD19 expression. Overall, this adoptive immunotherapy has already improved the lives of many with a previously incurable subset of ALL, and the future holds the promise of optimizing this treatment further.

References

1. Eshhar Z, Waks T, Gross G, Schindler DG (1993) Specific activation and targeting of cytotoxic lymphocytes through chimeric single chains consisting of antibody-binding domains and the gamma or zeta subunits of the immunoglobulin and T-cell receptors. Proc Natl Acad Sci U S A 90(2):720–724

2. June CH, O'Connor RS, Kawalekar OU, Ghassemi S, Milone MC (2018) CAR T cell immunotherapy for human cancer. Science 359(6382):1361–1365

3. Sadelain M (2015) CAR therapy: the CD19 paradigm. J Clin Invest 125(9):3392–3400

4. Kowolik CM, Topp MS, Gonzalez S, Pfeiffer T, Olivares S, Gonzalez N et al (2006) CD28 costimulation provided through a CD19-specific chimeric antigen receptor enhances in vivo persistence and antitumor efficacy of adoptively transferred T cells. Cancer Res 66 (22):10995–11004

5. Finney HM, Akbar AN, Lawson AD (2004) Activation of resting human primary T cells with chimeric receptors: costimulation from CD28, inducible costimulator, CD134, and CD137 in series with signals from the TCR zeta chain. J Immunol 172(1):104–113

6. Loskog A, Giandomenico V, Rossig C, Pule M, Dotti G, Brenner MK (2006) Addition of the CD28 signaling domain to chimeric T-cell receptors enhances chimeric T-cell resistance to T regulatory cells. Leukemia 20(10):1819–1828

7. Maher J, Brentjens RJ, Gunset G, Riviere I, Sadelain M (2002) Human T-lymphocyte cytotoxicity and proliferation directed by a single chimeric TCRzeta /CD28 receptor. Nat Biotechnol 20(1):70–75

8. Savoldo B, Ramos CA, Liu E, Mims MP, Keating MJ, Carrum G et al (2011) CD28 costimulation improves expansion and persistence of chimeric antigen receptor-modified T cells in lymphoma patients. J Clin Invest 121(5):1822–1826

9. Tammana S, Huang X, Wong M, Milone MC, Ma L, Levine BL et al (2010) 4–1BB and CD28 signaling plays a synergistic role in redirecting umbilical cord blood T cells against B-cell malignancies. Hum Gene Ther 21(1):75–86

10. Wang J, Jensen M, Lin Y, Sui X, Chen E, Lindgren CG et al (2007) Optimizing adoptive polyclonal T cell immunotherapy of lymphomas, using a chimeric T cell receptor possessing CD28 and CD137 costimulatory domains. Hum Gene Ther 18(8):712–725

11. FDA Approval

12. Kenderian SS, Ruella M, Gill S, Kalos M (2014) Chimeric antigen receptor T-cell therapy to target hematologic malignancies. Cancer Res 74(22):6383–6389

13. Kochenderfer JN (2014) Genetic engineering of T cells in leukemia and lymphoma. Clin Adv Hematol Oncol 12(3):190–192

14. Maus MV, Grupp SA, Porter DL, June CH (2014) Antibody-modified T cells: CARs take the front seat for hematologic malignancies. Blood 123(17):2625–2635

15. Sadelain M, Brentjens R, Riviere I (2013) The basic principles of chimeric antigen receptor design. Cancer Discov 3(4):388–398

16. Gill S, June CH (2015) Going viral: chimeric antigen receptor T-cell therapy for hematological malignancies. Immunol Rev 263(1):68–89

17. Turtle CJ, Hanafi LA, Berger C, Gooley TA, Cherian S, Hudecek M et al (2016) CD19 CAR-T cells of defined CD4+:CD8+ composition in adult B cell ALL patients. J Clin Invest 126(6):2123–2138

18. Hay KA, Gauthier J, Hirayama AV, Voutsinas JM, Wu Q, Li D et al (2019) Factors associated with durable EFS in adult B-cell ALL patients achieving MRD-negative CR after CD19 CAR T-cell therapy. Blood 133(15):1652–1663

19. Turtle CJ, Hanafi LA, Berger C, Daniel Sommermeyer P, Barbara Pender MS, Emily M, Robinson BS, Melville K et al (2015) Addition of fludarabine to cyclophosphamide lymphodepletion improves in vivo expansion of CD19 chimeric antigen receptor-modified T cells and clinical outcome in adults with B cell acute lymphoblastic leukemia. Blood 126 (23):3773

20. Gust J, Hay KA, Hanafi LA, Li D, Myerson D, Gonzalez-Cuyar LF et al (2017) Endothelial activation and blood-brain barrier disruption in neurotoxicity after adoptive immunotherapy with CD19 CAR-T cells. Cancer Discov 7(12):1404–1419

21. Park JH, Santomasso B, Riviere I, Senechal B, Wang X, Purdon T et al (2017) Baseline and early post-treatment clinical and laboratory factors associated with severe neurotoxicity following 19–28z CAR T cells in adult patients with relapsed B-ALL. J Clin Oncol 35:7024

22. Hay KA, Hanafi LA, Li D, Gust J, Liles WC, Wurfel MM et al (2017) Kinetics and biomarkers of severe cytokine release syndrome after CD19 chimeric antigen receptor-modified T-cell therapy. Blood 130(21):2295–2306

23. Brentjens RJ, Davila ML, Riviere I, Park J, Wang X, Cowell LG et al (2013) CD19-targeted T cells rapidly induce molecular remissions in adults with chemotherapy-refractory acute lymphoblastic leukemia. Sci Transl Med 5(177):177ra38

24. Brudno JN, Somerville RP, Shi V, Rose JJ, Halverson DC, Fowler DH et al (2016) Allogeneic T cells that express an anti-CD19 chimeric antigen receptor induce remissions of B-cell malignancies that progress after allogeneic hematopoietic stem-cell transplantation without causing graft-versus-host disease. J Clin Oncol 34(10):1112–1121

25. Cruz CR, Micklethwaite KP, Savoldo B, Ramos CA, Lam S, Ku S et al (2013) Infusion of donor-derived CD19-redirected virus-specific T cells for B-cell malignancies relapsed after allogeneic stem cell transplant: a phase 1 study. Blood 122(17):2965–2973

26. Davila ML, Riviere I, Wang X, Bartido S, Park J, Curran K et al (2014) Efficacy and toxicity management of 19–28z CAR T cell therapy in B cell acute lymphoblastic leukemia. Sci Transl Med 6(224):224ra25

27. Grupp SA, Kalos M, Barrett D, Aplenc R, Porter DL, Rheingold SR et al (2013) Chimeric antigen receptor-modified T cells for acute lymphoid leukemia. N Engl J Med 368(16):1509–1518

28. Lee DW, Kochenderfer JN, Stetler-Stevenson M, Cui YK, Delbrook C, Feldman SA et al (2015) T cells expressing CD19 chimeric antigen receptors for acute lymphoblastic leukaemia in children and young adults: a phase 1 dose-escalation trial. Lancet 385(9967):517–528

29. Park JH, Riviere I, Gonen M, Wang X, Senechal B, Curran KJ et al (2018) Long-term follow-up of CD19 CAR therapy in acute lymphoblastic leukemia. N Engl J Med 378(5):449–459

30. Maude SL, Laetsch TW, Buechner J, Rives S, Boyer M, Bittencourt H et al (2018) Tisagenlecleucel in children and young adults with B-cell lymphoblastic leukemia. N Engl J Med 378(5):439–448

31. Dong L, Chang LJ, Zhiyong G, Lu DP, Zhang JP, Wang JB et al (2015) Chimeric antigen receptor 4SCAR19-modified T cells in acute lymphoid leukemia: a phase II multi-center clinical trial in China. Blood 126(23):3774

32. Maude SL, Frey N, Shaw PA, Aplenc R, Barrett DM, Bunin NJ et al (2014) Chimeric antigen receptor T cells for sustained remissions in leukemia. N Engl J Med 371(16):1507–1517

33. Rheingold SR, Chen LL, Maude SL, Aplenc R, Barker C, Barrett DM et al (2015) Efficient trafficking of chimeric antigen receptor (CAR)-modified T cells to CSF and induction of durable CNS remissions in children with CNS/combined relapsed/refractory ALL. Blood 126 (23):3769

34. Jacoby E, Bielorai B, Avigdor A, Itzhaki O, Hutt D, Nussboim V et al (2018) Locally produced CD19 CAR T cells leading to clinical remissions in medullary and extramedullary relapsed acute lymphoblastic leukemia. Am J Hematol 93(12):1485–1492

35. Zhang H, Hu Y, Wei G, Wu W, Huang H (2019) Successful chimeric antigen receptor T cells therapy in extramedullary relapses of acute lymphoblastic leukemia after allogeneic hematopoietic stem cell transplantation. Bone Marrow Transplant

36. Wang D, Shi R, Wang Q, Li J (2018) Extramedullary relapse of acute lymphoblastic leukemia after allogeneic hematopoietic stem cell transplantation treated by CAR T-cell therapy: a case report. Onco Targets Ther 11:6327–6332

37. Lee DW, Santomasso BD, Locke FL, Ghobadi A, Turtle CJ, Brudno JN et al (2019) ASTCT consensus grading for cytokine release syndrome and neurologic toxicity associated with immune effector cells. Biol Blood Marrow Transplant 25(4):625–638

38. Chang LJ, Dong L, Liu YC, Tsao ST, Li YC, Liu L et al (2016) Safety and efficacy evaluation of 4SCAR19 chimeric antigen receptor-modified T cells targeting B cell acute lymphoblastic leukemia—three-year follow-up of a multicenter phase I/II study. Blood 128(22):587

39. Pan J, Yang JF, Deng BP, Zhao XJ, Zhang X, Lin YH et al (2017) High efficacy and safety of low-dose CD19-directed CAR-T cell therapy in 51 refractory or relapsed B acute lymphoblastic leukemia patients. Leukemia 31(12):2587–2593

40. National Cancer Institute. Common terminology criteria for adverse events v4.3 (CTCAE)

41. National Cancer Institute. Common terminology criteria for adverse events (CTCAE). Version 5.0

42. Lee DW, Gardner R, Porter DL, Louis CU, Ahmed N, Jensen M et al (2014) Current concepts in the diagnosis and management of cytokine release syndrome. Blood 124(2):188–195

43. Neelapu SS, Tummala S, Kebriaei P, Wierda W, Gutierrez C, Locke FL et al (2018) Chimeric antigen receptor T-cell therapy—assessment and management of toxicities. Nat Rev Clin Oncol 15(1):47–62

44. Porter D, Frey N, Wood PA, Weng Y, Grupp SA (2018) Grading of cytokine release syndrome associated with the CAR T cell therapy tisagenlecleucel. J Hematol Oncol 11(1):35

45. Titov A, Petukhov A, Staliarova A, Motorin D, Bulatov E, Shuvalov O et al (2018) The biological basis and clinical symptoms of CAR-T therapy-associated toxicites. Cell Death Dis 9(9):897

46. Teachey DT, Lacey SF, Shaw PA, Melenhorst JJ, Maude SL, Frey N et al (2016) Identification of predictive biomarkers for cytokine release syndrome after chimeric antigen receptor T-cell therapy for acute lymphoblastic leukemia. Cancer Discov 6(6):664–679

47. Porter DL, Hwang WT, Frey NV, Lacey SF, Shaw PA, Loren AW et al (2015) Chimeric antigen receptor T cells persist and induce sustained remissions in relapsed refractory chronic lymphocytic leukemia. Sci Transl Med 7(303):303ra139

48. Kalos M, Levine BL, Porter DL, Katz S, Grupp SA, Bagg A et al (2011) T cells with chimeric antigen receptors have potent antitumor effects and can establish memory in patients with advanced leukemia. Sci Transl Med 3(95):95ra73

49. Chen F, Teachey DT, Pequignot E, Frey N, Porter D, Maude SL et al (2016) Measuring IL-6 and sIL-6R in serum from patients treated with tocilizumab and/or siltuximab following CAR T cell therapy. J Immunol Methods 434:1–8

50. Hu Y, Sun J, Wu Z, Yu J, Cui Q, Pu C et al (2016) Predominant cerebral cytokine release syndrome in CD19-directed chimeric antigen receptor-modified T cell therapy. J Hematol Oncol 9(1):70

51. Abramson JS, McGree B, Noyes S, Plummer S, Wong C, Chen YB et al (2017) Anti-CD19 CAR T cells in CNS diffuse large-B-cell lymphoma. N Engl J Med 377(8):783–784

52. van der Heyde HC, Nolan J, Combes V, Gramaglia I, Grau GE (2006) A unified hypothesis for the genesis of cerebral malaria: sequestration, inflammation and hemostasis leading to microcirculatory dysfunction. Trends Parasitol 22(11):503–508

53. Grau GE, Heremans H, Piguet PF, Pointaire P, Lambert PH, Billiau A et al (1989) Monoclonal antibody against interferon gamma can prevent experimental cerebral malaria and its associated overproduction of tumor necrosis factor. Proc Natl Acad Sci U S A 86 (14):5572–5574

54. Danylesko I, Chowers G, Shouval R, Besser MJ, Jacoby E, Shimoni A et al (2019) Treatment with anti CD19 chimeric antigen receptor T cells after antibody-based immunotherapy in adults with acute lymphoblastic leukemia. Curr Res Transl Med

55. Jacoby E (2019) The role of allogeneic HSCT after CAR T cells for acute lymphoblastic leukemia. Bone Marrow Transplant 54(Suppl 2):810–814

56. Kenderian SS, Porter DL, Gill S (2017) Chimeric antigen receptor T cells and hematopoietic cell transplantation: how not to put the CART before the horse. Biol Blood Marrow Transplant 23(2):235–246

57. Grupp SA, Maude SL, Shaw PA, Aplenc R, Barrett DM, Callahan C et al (2015) Durable remissions in children with relapsed/refractory ALL treated with T cells engineered with a CD19-targeted chimeric antigen receptor (CTL019). Blood 126(23):681

58. Fielding AK, Richards SM, Chopra R, Lazarus HM, Litzow MR, Buck G et al (2007) Outcome of 609 adults after relapse of acute lymphoblastic leukemia (ALL); an MRC UKALL12/ECOG 2993 study. Blood 109(3):944–950

59. Horowitz MM, Gale RP, Sondel PM, Goldman JM, Kersey J, Kolb HJ et al (1990) Graft-versus-leukemia reactions after bone marrow transplantation. Blood 75(3):555–562

60. Pulsipher MA, Langholz B, Wall DA, Schultz KR, Bunin N, Carroll WL et al (2014) The addition of sirolimus to tacrolimus/methotrexate GVHD prophylaxis in children with ALL: a phase 3 children's oncology group/pediatric blood and marrow transplant consortium trial. Blood 123(13):2017–2025

61. Bader P, Kreyenberg H, Henze GH, Eckert C, Reising M, Willasch A et al (2009) Prognostic value of minimal residual disease quantification before allogeneic stem-cell transplantation in relapsed childhood acute lymphoblastic leukemia: the ALL-REZ BFM study group. J Clin Oncol 27(3):377–384

62. Gardner RA, Finney O, Annesley C, Brakke H, Summers C, Leger K et al (2017) Intent-to-treat leukemia remission by CD19 CAR T cells of defined formulation and dose in children and young adults. Blood 129(25):3322–3331

63. Long AH, Haso WM, Shern JF, Wanhainen KM, Murgai M, Ingaramo M et al (2015) 4–1BB costimulation ameliorates T cell exhaustion induced by tonic signaling of chimeric antigen receptors. Nat Med 21(6):581–590

64. Milone MC, Fish JD, Carpenito C, Carroll RG, Binder GK, Teachey D et al (2009) Chimeric receptors containing CD137 signal transduction domains mediate enhanced survival of T cells and increased antileukemic efficacy in vivo. Mol Ther 17(8):1453–1464

65. Mejstrikova E, Hrusak O, Borowitz MJ, Whitlock JA, Brethon B, Trippett TM et al (2017) CD19-negative relapse of pediatric B-cell precursor acute lymphoblastic leukemia following blinatumomab treatment. Blood Cancer J 7(12):659

66. Sotillo E, Barrett DM, Black KL, Bagashev A, Oldridge D, Wu G et al (2015) Convergence of acquired mutations and alternative splicing of CD19 enables resistance to CART-19 immunotherapy. Cancer Discov 5(12):1282–1295

67. Fischer J, Paret C, El Malki K, Alt F, Wingerter A, Neu MA et al (2017) CD19 isoforms enabling resistance to CART-19 immunotherapy are expressed in B-ALL patients at initial diagnosis. J Immunother 40(5):187–195

68. Jacoby E, Nguyen SM, Fountaine TJ, Welp K, Gryder B, Qin H et al (2016) CD19 CAR immune pressure induces B-precursor acute lymphoblastic leukaemia lineage switch exposing inherent leukaemic plasticity. Nat Commun 7.12320

69. Gardner R, Wu D, Cherian S, Fang M, Hanafi LA, Finney O et al (2016) Acquisition of a CD19-negative myeloid phenotype allows immune escape of MLL-rearranged B-ALL from CD19 CAR-T-cell therapy. Blood 127(20):2406–2410

70. Mullighan CG, Phillips LA, Su X, Ma J, Miller CB, Shurtleff SA et al (2008) Genomic analysis of the clonal origins of relapsed acute lymphoblastic leukemia. Science 322 (5906):1377–1380

71. Rayes A, McMasters RL, O'Brien MM (2016) Lineage Switch in MLL-Rearranged infant leukemia following CD19-directed therapy. Pediatr Blood Cancer 63(6):1113–1115

72. Nagel I, Bartels M, Duell J, Oberg HH, Ussat S, Bruckmueller H et al (2017) Hematopoietic stem cell involvement in BCR-ABL1-positive ALL as a potential mechanism of resistance to blinatumomab therapy. Blood 130(18):2027–2031

73. Oberley MJ, Gaynon PS, Bhojwani D, Pulsipher MA, Gardner RA, Hiemenz MC et al (2018) Myeloid lineage switch following chimeric antigen receptor T-cell therapy in a patient with

TCF3-ZNF384 fusion-positive B-lymphoblastic leukemia. Pediatr Blood Cancer 65(9): e27265

74. Lee DW, Stetler-Stevenson M, Yuan C, Shah NN, Delbrook C, Yates B et al (2016) Long-term outcomes following CD19 CAR T cell therapy for B-ALL are superior in patients receiving a fludarabine/cyclophosphamide preparative regimen and post-car hematopoietic stem cell transplantation. Blood 128(22):218

75. Zhang Y, Chen H, Song Y, Tan X, Zhao Y, Liu X et al (2019) Post-chimeric antigen receptor T-cell therapy haematopoietic stem cell transplantation for 52 cases with refractory/relapsed B-cell acute lymphoblastic leukaemia. Br J Haematol

Printed in the United States
by Baker & Taylor Publisher Services